4 weeks to better sleep

A life-changing plan for deep sleep, improved brain function and feeling great

DR MICHAEL MOSLEY

SIMON &
SCHUSTER

London · New York · Sydney · Toronto · New Delhi

4 WEEKS TO BETTER SLEEP
First published in Australia in 2024 by
Simon & Schuster (Australia) Pty Limited
Suite 19A, Level 1, Building C, 450 Miller Street, Cammeray, NSW 2062
First published in 2020 by Short Books as *Fast Asleep*
an imprint of Octopus Publishing Group Ltd, an Hachette UK Company
10 9 8 7 6 5 4 3 2 1

Simon & Schuster: Celebrating 100 Years of Publishing in 2024.
Sydney New York London Toronto New Delhi
Visit our website at www.simonandschuster.com.au

 A catalogue record for this book is available from the National Library of Australia

ISBN: 9781761425929
Illustrations: E.K. Mosley
Cover design: Mel Four
Photography: Smith & Gilmour
Food Styling: Phil Mundy
Typesetting: Jeremy Tilson
Back cover photograph © David Bostock
Cover text and design © Hachette UK Ltd

Printed and bound in Australia by Griffin Press

Contents

Introduction   1

Part One: The Science of Sleep

1. How we woke up to sleep   17

2. What puts us to sleep   45

3. What keeps us awake   57

4. Are you getting enough?   87

5. Tried and tested ways to boost your sleep   109

6. Eating your way to a good night's sleep   141

Part Two: The 4-Week Sleep Plan

7. The plan in practice   171

8. Goodnight from me   221

Recipes by Dr Clare Bailey and Justine Pattison   223

Endnotes   293

Index   300

Acknowledgements   315

About the authors   316

Introduction

Sleep is something we all do; in fact, we spend around a third of our lives in this strange, unconscious state. And yet until recently we understood very little about what sleep is for, how much we need, and the role that dreams play in improving our mental health.

The good news is that over the last 20 years there has been a revolution in our understanding of sleep and just how important it is. Not so long ago it was fashionable to brag that you hardly slept at all, and the mark of a successful business person or politician was their ability to get by on very little shut-eye. Former British Prime Minister Margaret Thatcher was held up as a shining example of someone who could operate without much sleep (which turned out to be a carefully cultivated myth), while I remember being told by a grizzled medical consultant, when I complained about the impact that lack of sleep was having on my empathy and judgement, that 'sleep is for wimps'. Or, as another put it: 'There's plenty of time to sleep when you are dead.'

Our current attitudes to sleep are very different. Thanks to recent research, we know that too little sleep can devastate your body, brain and microbiome (gut bacteria), dramatically increasing your risk of developing a range of chronic conditions such as obesity, type 2 diabetes and dementia.

And, when it comes to sleep, it's not just about quantity, but about quality too. We have learned, through extensive sleep studies, that if you don't get enough of the right sort of sleep, you increase your risk of depression and memory problems. Which is all very worrying, particularly if, like a third of the adult population, you suffer from insomnia.

Fortunately, there are surprising and highly effective ways to improve your sleep quality, ensuring you fall asleep rapidly, get plenty of deep sleep and wake up feeling refreshed. This in turn should boost your happiness, creativity and even life expectancy.

The reason I particularly wanted to write this book is because I am obsessed by sleep and have been for many years, not just from a science perspective, but also on a deeply personal level. I have lots of friends who suffer from insomnia and for the last 20 years, I have also suffered quite badly from intermittent insomnia, to the point where I was in real despair. I wanted to find out what I was doing wrong and, of course, I wanted to find out what I could do to make it better.

I wasn't always a poor sleeper. When I was a teenager, I could sleep any time, anywhere. I once slept in a photo booth (I had missed the last train home). Another time I slept in a telephone kiosk. I never worried about going to sleep or staying asleep, because that came naturally.

I didn't always get a good night's sleep, but that was my choice. Like most teenagers, I was keen to burn the candle at both ends. As a medical student, I often stayed up partying, then went straight into some feverish last-minute cramming. Which I now realise was wildly counterproductive. You need sleep to consolidate your memories, as I will explain in this book.

As my medical training progressed, sleep became ever more precious. I found I just couldn't function any longer on a few hours' sleep a night. I became intensely irritable and I'm sure that both my judgement and my empathy were impaired. But, even so, I could still go to sleep and stay deeply asleep for hours when I was given the chance. Despite the disruption to my sleep pattern caused by the irregular hours I had to work, I never had any problem drifting off.

Then, as I entered my late twenties, everything changed. By then I was married and I had started a new career in television. The hours were long and unpredictable, though nothing like as bad as in medicine. At this time my wife, Clare, was working as a junior doctor and regularly working 120 hours a week. It was not unusual for her to be on duty for three or four days with only a few hours of broken sleep a night, which blunted her thinking. She told me that after one particularly gruelling week, she briefly fell asleep standing, during an operation. Fortunately, she woke up before anyone noticed.

Not only did work absorb almost every waking hour, it also began to intrude on our sleep. On the occasions that Clare was actually sleeping at home, she would regularly wake me up in the middle of the night to help her look for patients, which in her sleep-deprived state she was convinced were lost in the cupboards or waiting for her downstairs. Clare has parasomnia, a quite common set of sometimes bizarre nocturnal behaviours, which include a tendency towards sleepwalking and sleep talking.

By the early 1990s, we had started to have children, and that, of course, resulted in many nights of disrupted sleep. In fact, we went on to have four children, which meant that a full decade was dominated by babies.

By the time we entered our forties, Clare was a GP and working more regular hours. Our children were also sleeping through the night. But by then I had begun to show classic signs of insomnia. I had difficulty going to sleep and kept waking up at three in the morning with thoughts rushing through my head. I would lie there for what felt like hours, and going to bed, which was once a real pleasure, was something I began to approach with a sense of unease. Would this be a good night or a bad night? Would I get up feeling shattered or would this be one of those rare nights when I would sleep through until morning?

Naturally enough, I wanted to understand what was going on and what I could do to get back to the days of blissful, effortless sleep. I made what was to be the first of many popular television programmes examining the mystery of sleep. Making these programmes introduced me to lots of sleep scientists and a whole new, fascinating world of sleep research.

To try and understand the impact of severe sleep deprivation, I decided to see how long I could stay awake with a man who holds the unofficial world record. He can go days on end with no sleep at all, without appearing to suffer. What was the secret to his success? Why could he just keep going, while I couldn't?

Since then, I have interviewed hundreds of people, ranging from sleep experts to firefighters, doctors, astronauts and police officers, about their sleep. But the thing that really changed my sleeping life was a television series I made called *Australia's Sleep Revolution*.

Australia's Sleep Revolution

As part of my quest to learn more about sleep in general, and my own sleep in particular, in 2023 I agreed to present a three-part television series for the wonderful SBS (Special Broadcasting Service), called *Australia's Sleep Revolution*.

The idea behind the series, which first went out on Australian television in early 2024, is that I would take part in a clinical trial run by experts from Flinders University Sleep Institute in Adelaide. What made this trail so unusual, and from my perspective, so compelling, is that it combined a personalised approach with cutting edge sleep monitoring technology.

I knew that I was in good hands because, when it comes to sleep, the Flinders team are truly world class. They include sleep and respiratory doctors, psychologists, biomedical engineers, physiologists and even a dentist (who turned out to be particularly important for me).

Working with a television production company called Artemis Media (who I really rate), the Flinders team agreed to use their expertise to try and sort out the sleep problems of thirty people, and do it in just 8 weeks.

When I'm making a documentary I love getting stuck in, so naturally enough I agreed to be one of thirty volunteers. To be honest I was rather nervous about this as I wasn't sure what they would find. But despite my initial fears it was one of the best things I have ever done, both personally and professionally. And I do think the series, as well as changing the lives of many of the participants, also has the potential to change attitudes to treating sleep problems in Australia, and more widely.

The first thing I did was meet the team, led by Professor Danny Eckert, who explained to me what would happen over the next 8 weeks and what they hoped to achieve. Another key member of the team, and someone who supported me every step of the way, is Dr Sutapa Mukherjee, a leading sleep physician and a tireless sleep campaigner.

I also met a number of the volunteers who were about to take part in the trial. They came from every walk of life but what they had in common was they suffered from a range of chronic but very common sleep disorders, and many had forgotten what it was like to have a good night's sleep.

One of those volunteers was Priyanka, a young working mother who told me she was surviving on close to half the recommended amount of sleep. Her problem was that she would go to bed with her husband at a reasonable hour but, while he promptly went to sleep, she would lie awake for many hours, before eventually falling asleep sometime in the early hours of the morning. Then, around 6am, she'd be woken by the alarm going off, the start of her working day. As a result, she was feeling extremely sleep deprived, and on edge, 'My husband thinks it's a superpower', she said, 'that I can still function with 3- or 4-hours sleep. But he notices my irritability. I get angry a bit quickly if I'm not well rested.'

Like all the other participants in the trial I started off by having a medical examination, to exclude any health problems. I was then given some kit to take home, including a couple of different sleep trackers and something called a Withings Sleep Analyzer mat, which you can buy online and contains, amongst other things, a microphone. The idea is you slip it under your mattress, and it detects the breathing sounds and movements that you make while you are sleeping. You sync it to a smart phone and the next morning it will tell you how well you slept, whether you snored and whether you might have sleep apnoea. With our consent, data from all these devices were sent to the Flinders team. We were also all given a sleep diary to fill in, as that is a key part of the programme.

More surprisingly, I was given an electronic pill to swallow, linked by Bluetooth to a recording device. As psychologist Professor Leon Lack explained, the pill is a very accurate way of measuring core body temperature, the temperature of your internal organs. The reason this matters is because your core body temperature is, like so many other processes in our bodies, driven by our internal, circadian clock and is linked to sleep. Core body temperature changes across the course of a day, but should be at its lowest around 4am, which helps us stay asleep for the second half of the night. The Flinders team wanted to see if any of us had circadian clocks that were out of sync, either running faster or slower than you might expect which can lead to sleep disruption and symptoms of insomnia.

This used to be measured using a rectal thermometer, which had to be kept in place, so I was grateful that I was only required to swallow a pill.

After a few days getting acclimatised to all this kit, I went into the Nick Antic Flinders Sleep Laboratory for an overnight assessment. This involved having electrodes attached to my head and body, along with other devices to monitor me while I slept. It wasn't the best night's sleep I've had, but it was oddly reassuring to know that everyone else in the study was going through the same thing.

So, after all that monitoring, what did they find?

To be honest, it was a bit of a shock. They told me that I had quite severe insomnia, which I knew, but that I also had obstructive sleep apnoea (where you regularly stop breathing during the night – more on that on page 63). Sleep apnoea could explain why I often felt shattered during the day. They also said that I had a body clock which runs faster than expected. So, while most people's core body temperature (which is linked to the body clock) is at its lowest around 4am, and then starts to rise, the temperature-measuring pills I'd been swallowing showed that mine was at its lowest around 1am. That in turn could explain why I get so sleepy early in the evening and why I often wake up, feeling surprisingly alert, around 3.30am. In fact, Professor Lack said he thought my fast-running body clock could be what had triggered my insomnia in the first place (more on that on page 51).

It turned out that Priyanka had the opposite problem to me. They discovered her core body temperature dipped to its lowest point at around 6am, which explained why she found it so hard to go to sleep at a more normal hour, and why she found it so difficult to wake in the mornings.

To treat our circadian problems, we were both prescribed exposure to bright light, delivered by something called Re-Timer Light Therapy Glasses, developed by Professor Lack. The set I was given looks like a pair of white plastic-framed goggles, which fit over my glasses, and which shines a blue-enriched light into my eyes. It was odd wearing them around the house, to start with, but you get used to them. Priyanka was told to wear hers first thing in the morning, to try and bring her body clock earlier, while I was asked to wear mine in the evening, to push my body clock back. She was also encouraged to go out for early morning walks, while I was told to get more light in the evenings.

And it worked. Within a few weeks the tests on my core temperature showed that my body clock had shifted two hours later, while Priyanka, the extreme Owl, found that exposure to early morning light had the opposite effect, making it easier for her to fall asleep at night. As she later told me, 'It's been life changing... I am able to wake up without feeling like I'm fighting my body, and I'm ready to start off my day in a very, very positive mindset.' To find out more about light therapy and how to use it, see page 55.

To treat our underlying insomnia, a number of us, taking part in the trial were prescribed Sleep Restriction Therapy (SRT), which is also known as Bedtime Restriction Therapy. It is called that because, at least for a while, you are expected to cut back on the amount of time you spend in bed.

It might appear paradoxical to ask people who are suffering from insomnia to spend less time trying to sleep, but one of the classic mistakes people who have problems sleeping make is to spend more time in bed – when, for most people, lying in bed not sleeping isn't restful, it is very stressful. It also sets up a bad behaviour pattern where your brain comes to associate being in bed with being awake, fretting.

Studies have shown that bedtime restriction can be highly effective and long lasting. For me this meant, at least initially, going to bed at 11pm and getting up each morning at 5am. It was quite brutal to start with, but in combination with getting more evening light, I was soon sleeping better than I had for a long time. And once my sleep started to improve, which it did fairly fast, I was allowed a bit more time in bed each night, which was wonderful. By the end of the 8-week study I was declared insomnia free. More on bedtime restriction therapy and how to do it in a moment.

And as for the sleep apnoea, the team suggested that I might benefit from a twin pronged approach. I was given a device to strap round my neck, which looked a bit like a dog collar, but which contained a sensor that could tell when I was sleeping on my back and give me a little buzz, just enough to nudge me back to sleeping on my side. As well as that, the team dentist fitted me with a mandibular advancement device, a mouthguard which I was told to wear at night. It moves your lower jaw forward and stops your tongue falling back and blocking your airways. It was uncomfortable to start with, but within a few weeks tests showed that they were having an impact; I no longer had sleep apnoea. More on anti-snoring devices on page 66.

Getting a proper diagnosis, and treatments that really worked, was a massive relief, but also bittersweet. My dad died at the age of 74 of heart failure and it's obvious to me now, that as well as type 2 diabetes he must have had sleep apnoea, which contributed to his early death. And that makes me sad because if he had been diagnosed he could have been treated and he might still be with us.

As for the Flinders sleep treatment trial, the results were outstanding. Thirty people began the trial with a range of sleep problems, including chronic insomnia, sleep apnoea or both. Many had failed to find help in the past, yet with the help of light therapy, CBTi (cognitive behavioural therapy for insomnia, which can include sleep restriction therapy) and the judicious use of various sleep apnoea treatments, the multidisciplinary team at Flinders were able to successfully treat over 80% of the participants.

The structure of the book

You may be someone who is desperate to get a good night's sleep. Or you may simply be interested in what happens to you when your eyes close and you drift off into the land of Nod.

The first part of this book is all about the science of sleep: the research that has led to our current knowledge and how this has given us rich insights into a previously undiscovered land. What are common sleep disorders and how do they arise? What really happens to your brain and body when they are chronically sleep deprived? Why are dreams so important and how can you make the most of them?

I will use my own sleep adventures to illuminate the journey and I will, of course, provide plenty of scientific studies to justify my more surprising claims.

All of this lays the groundwork for the second part of the book, which is primarily aimed at helping you sleep better.

4 weeks to better sleep

As the title of the book suggests, I will take you through a sleep plan that should, within a few weeks, set you on a better path. As part of that I will share with you, in greater detail, some of the strategies used in *Australia's Sleep Revolution*.

No book can hope to replicate what the Flinders team managed to achieve, and if you have severe sleep problems then I would strongly recommend that you try to get referred to a sleep specialist.

That said, I am hopeful that if you follow the advice in this book it will make a significant difference to how well you sleep. Do also bear in mind that though I have labelled this as a 4-week programme, for some it will take longer to have an impact. And if you are to improve your sleep long term, it is also important that you incorporate into your everyday life at least some of the elements of sleep hygiene, stress management and a healthier lifestyle that I will be describing in a moment.

So where do you begin? A good place to start is to first identify why you are sleeping badly. You might think this is obvious – it's because you are stressed and anxious, with thoughts flying around your head when you go to bed, worrying about all the little things on your to-do list or grappling with big questions about your life's direction. Or perhaps it's because you wake up in the middle of the night, needing to go to the loo and you find that you struggle to doze off afterwards.

But when it comes to sleep, the most obvious cause isn't necessarily the right one. It could be that the reason why you feel stressed and anxious is because of your diet, or perhaps it is lack of sleep that is making you stressed and anxious, rather than the other way round. I have met a lot of people whose psychological problems almost entirely disappeared once they had got on top of their sleep.

In the course of looking at solutions for your sleep problems, I'm going to introduce you to Sleep Apnoea, Sleep Hygiene, Bright Light Therapy, Sleep Restriction Therapy and the concept of 'sleep efficiency'.

In fact, one of my key goals is to help you improve your 'sleep efficiency', which is a measure of how well you've slept. After all, the main complaint people have about their sleep is that they spend far too much of the night tossing and turning, unable to sleep.

Quality is at least as important and quantity, and if you are spending much of the night in bed, failing to sleep (and fearing the consequences for your brain and body of not falling asleep) then that is going to be upsetting.

So, your sleep efficiency is a key measure. It represents the amount of time you spend in bed asleep, as opposed to trying to get to sleep or lying in bed wide awake, fretting. You should be aiming for a sleep efficiency of 85%. More on that later.

As well as all of the above, I also want to help you improve your sleep by improving your diet. Forget all those stories about turkey or cheese. It turns out that eating more legumes and fibre-rich foods, and fewer late-night sugary snacks, is one of the most effective ways to boost your levels of deep sleep and improve your mood.

That's, in part, because fibre-rich foods feed the trillions of 'good' bacteria that live in your gut, which in turn produce chemicals that have been shown to reduce stress and anxiety. I will take you on a fascinating guided tour of the science.

On a more practical level, my wife Clare, along with food writer Justine Pattison, has created a range of tasty recipes that are packed with the sorts of ingredients that those good bacteria will really love, and that you will love too.

I do hope you enjoy this book and most of all I hope it puts you to sleep. Fast.

PART ONE:
The Science of Sleep

1. How we woke up to sleep

As I pointed out in my introduction, it is astonishing that despite the fact that we spend up to a third of our lives – around 25 years – asleep, until relatively recently we knew very little about what went on during that time. A hundred years ago, most people thought that the brain simply switched off, like a light bulb, when you went to sleep.

The American inventor Thomas Edison, who manufactured the first light bulbs, and whose invention did more than any other to disrupt our sleeping patterns, thought that sleep was a waste of time. He claimed to need less than five hours' sleep a night and said that having more was just greedy. As he put it: 'Most people overeat 100%, and oversleep 100%, because they like it. That extra 100% makes them unhealthy and inefficient.'

As we'll see, he couldn't have been more wrong. One reason we knew so little about sleep was that until the early 20th century we had no means to probe it. Scientists like being able to measure things, and sleep was all too intangible. It was like trying to make sense of the movements of the planets before we had the ability to properly study the heavens.

The man who made the first major breakthrough in the science of sleep was a peculiar German psychiatrist called Hans Berger.

Reading the sleeping mind

Hans Berger's contribution was the invention of electroencephalography (often abbreviated to EEG), the ability to record human 'brainwaves' by attaching electrodes to a volunteer's skull.

He built the first working electroencephalograph in 1924, but for a long time his work was ignored. He was widely regarded as a crank. And that's not surprising because Berger believed passionately in telepathy. In fact, the main reason he had created his EEG machine was to prove that humans can communicate with each other through psychic powers.

His obsession with telepathy began when he was a young cavalry officer. One day, while he was taking part in a military exercise, his horse suddenly reared and threw him into the path of a horse-drawn cannon. He wasn't seriously injured, but he was very shaken. He later discovered that his sister, who was at home at the time, had had a sudden premonition that he was in deadly danger and forced their father to send him a telegram to see if he was alright.

Berger was convinced that during the accident, he had sent out a powerful psychic distress message, which his sister had somehow picked up. He was so convinced of this that he decided to retrain as a doctor, and then as a psychiatrist, just to prove that telepathy exists.

I personally don't believe in telepathy, but Berger was absolutely right when he claimed that the human brain produces electrical signals that can be 'read' by multiple electrodes placed on the scalp. Although modern versions of the EEG are far more sophisticated than Berger's invention, in essence they do the same thing.

Dream sleep

Berger had shown, in 1924, that his EEG machine could be used to study human brainwaves, but it would be another 27 years before sleep researchers got round to using it in any meaningful way.

In December 1951, an impoverished student at the University of Chicago called Eugene Aserinsky decided to take his eight-year-old son, Armond, to his lab to take part in a novel sleep experiment. He scrubbed Armond's scalp, taped on the EEG electrodes and left him to fall asleep. Aserinsky then went next door to record what happened.

For Aserinsky this was a do-or-die moment. He was 30 years old and living with his newly pregnant wife in a converted army barracks. They were so poor he could barely afford the HP payments on his typewriter, let alone heat their home. He needed a breakthrough with his research, and soon.

Since no one else had yet bothered to use an EEG to study someone sleeping through an entire night, Aserinsky had decided he might as well begin with his young son.

Nothing very exciting happened for the first hour, but then he noticed that his machine had begun to record a sudden change in brain activity. On the machine, it looked as if his son Armond had woken up. But when Aserinsky went next door to check, Armond was clearly still deeply asleep. Nothing was moving except for his eyes, which were darting around under his eyelids.

Aserinsky woke the boy, who reported that he had been having an intense dream. This was amazing, ground-breaking stuff. The next day Eugene repeated the experiment, with the same results. A few hours after Armond fell asleep, the EEG recorded a sudden change in his brain activity, which coincided with rapid eye movements. Studies done with other, adult, volunteers showed the same thing.

Eugene Aserinsky had done something that would transform our understanding of sleep. He had sent the first exploratory probes into Planet Sleep and discovered that, far from being a dull, barren world where not much happens, it is a place where the brain undergoes some remarkable changes. Sleep research was about to become sexy.

However, despite having made this amazing breakthrough, Aserinsky soon lost interest in sleep. After publishing his findings in 1954, he went off to study electrical brain activity in salmon and later died in a car crash, very possibly because he fell asleep at the wheel.

So what does happen when we sleep?

I've spent many nights both being observed in sleep labs and, more interestingly, observing other people while they sleep. If you have never seen someone else go to sleep, or had yourself filmed while falling asleep, then I would recommend you give it a go. It is very entertaining.

As I mentioned earlier, we used to think of going to sleep as being like switching off a light bulb. You were either awake or asleep. We now know it is much more complicated than that.

Sleep involves three distinct states: light sleep, deep sleep and REM (Rapid Eye Movement) sleep. We sleep in roughly 90-minute cycles throughout the night, flipping between one state and another.

As you can see from the diagram below, during the first part of the night you get most of your deep sleep, while the second half of the night is dominated by REM sleep. Most people wake two or three times a night. If you are lucky (like my wife Clare), you won't even be aware of it. If you are unlucky, you will wake up and stay awake.

Hypnogram

When you go to bed and close your eyes, you should soon start to drift off into light sleep (Stage 1). At this point you are drowsy, but easy to rouse. If the dog next door starts to bark or your partner starts to snore loudly, you might wake up.

After Stage 1 (which normally lasts around 10 minutes), you begin a deeper dive into sleep.

When it comes to sleep, I like to see myself as a seal, plunging joyfully into the depths of the night. Some years ago, I made a film about free divers, people who swim to great depths without the aid of oxygen tanks, and it looked just beautiful, as they headed away from the bright light of the surface towards the dark of the ocean floor. That said, for some people, the act of falling asleep is frustrating rather than joyful.

The next stage, Stage 2, also counts as 'light sleep'. As you enter it, your core body temperature (typically measured with a rectal thermometer), which began to fall even before you got into bed, drops even further.

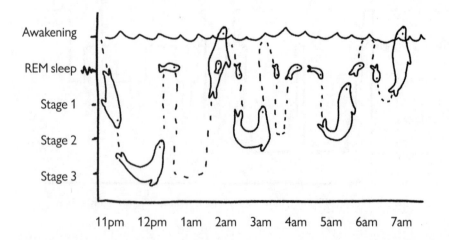

Your heart rate slows down (I've recorded mine and it drops from its usual 60 beats a minute to about 55) and your breathing also slows and becomes steadier.

When you are entering Stage 2, you may well do what is known as a hypnagogic jerk or 'sleep start'. This is an involuntary twitch of the muscles as you go deeper into sleep. Most of us do it. Although it is normally no more than a little twitch, some people really lash out, which is no fun if you are sharing a bed with them. It is often a sign of stress, and if you follow the regime I'm going to outline in this book, you should not only sleep better but also be less likely to do this annoying little dance at night.

If all is going well, within an hour of beginning to nod off you will have entered Stage 3 – deep sleep. This is also known as slow-wave sleep because it is when an EEG would start recording slow, deep waves. Millions of neurons in your brain fire at once, then pause, before firing again. This activity creates great, crashing waves that travel through the brain, which are really hypnotic to watch on a screen.

In deep sleep you are at your most relaxed and difficult to rouse. But, while your brain rests, your body is hard at work because deep sleep is when a lot of vital repair work gets done. Your pituitary gland, for example, will start to secrete more growth hormone, which is vital for cell growth and repair. Deep sleep also boosts your immune system.

Without sufficient deep sleep, your body makes fewer cytokines, a type of protein that regulates your immune system. Cytokines are vital for helping you fight infections, which is why lack of sleep makes you more vulnerable to catching colds and also reduces the efficacy of vaccines against diseases such as the flu.

In a recent paper, for example, researchers from the University of Chicago and the French National Institute of Health and Medicine looked at the results of seven studies where people had been vaccinated for viral infections like influenza and hepatitis. They found that people who slept for 6 hours or less a night produced a much weaker response to the vaccination than those who got 7–9 hours a night. So if you want your immune system to be in optimal condition to fight off infections, you do need to get at least 6 hours of sleep a night and preferably more.

Despite the fact that deep sleep is supposed to be a time of deep relaxation, it is also the time when some people start to do strange things, like sleepwalking, sleep talking and even sleep eating. I will talk about these phenomena in more detail in Chapter 3.

Deep sleep and brain cleaning

When I was young, I loved reading stories from Greek mythology and one of my heroes was the super powerful Heracles (known as Hercules by the Romans). Heracles, who was the son of Zeus, was told he could be made immortal if he successfully carried out 12 apparently impossible tasks ('the labours of Heracles').

The least glamorous of these challenges was to clean out the Augean stables, in a single night. The Augean stables were notorious because they housed more than 3000 cattle and hadn't been cleaned for years. You can just imagine the stink. Yet Heracles succeeded in scouring the stables of decades of accumulated dung, in the allotted time of a single night, by diverting two rivers through them.

The reason I bring up this story is that, overnight, something similar takes place inside your head. A network of channels in your brain, known as the glymphatic system, opens up and pumps cerebrospinal fluid through it while you are in deep sleep. Like the rivers in the Augean stables, this fluid flows through your brain tissue and washes away the toxic waste that has built up there during the day.

That's the good news. The bad news is that, as we get older, we tend to get less deep sleep, which means that our brains are not as good at washing away the toxins. Young people typically get a couple of hours of deep sleep a night. When you get to my age (66), you are lucky if you are getting 30 minutes.

This matters because it is the accumulation of toxic proteins in the brain, such as beta amyloid and tau, that appears to drive Alzheimer's disease, and in humans there is a very clear link between poor sleep and the development of dementia. Or another, more positive way of looking at this is that getting decent sleep can protect you against the risk of slowly losing your mind. There is even evidence that getting a good night's sleep can help people who are already at high risk of developing dementia slow down progression of the disease.

In a recent study, published in May 2023, researchers from UC Berkeley's Center for Human Sleep Science recruited 62 older adults to take part in a short trial. Before they started, the participants (who were all healthy adults without obvious signs of dementia), were asked to have a positron emission tomography (PET) scanner, to measure just how much beta-amyloid they had in their brains.

Many of them, despite appearing healthy, already had increased levels of beta-amyloid.

This group were asked to sleep in a lab while researchers monitored their sleep waves with an electroencephalography (EEG) machine.

After spending a closely monitored night's sleep in the lab, the participants were asked to do a memory task involving matching names to faces.

It turned out that despite having high amounts of beta-amyloid deposits in their brain, the people who had managed to get lots of deep sleep performed better than expected in the memory test, and far better than the volunteers with the same amount of amyloid deposits, but who had slept worse.

The researchers say this adds to existing evidence that deep, slow-wave sleep can help protect your brain, and especially your memory, even if you already have a build-up of toxins in your brain. As one of them put it, you can think of deep sleep as being like a life raft, keeping your memory afloat, while the toxins try to drag it down into the watery depths of Alzheimer's disease.[1]

To maximise your chance of getting more deep sleep, it is essential that you stick to a regular sleep schedule, stay mentally and physically active during the day, create a cool and dark sleep environment and minimise screen time before bed. A warm shower before turning in for the night has also been shown to increase the quality of deep, slow-wave sleep. And do try to get to bed before midnight, since your brain gets the most deep sleep during the first half of the night.

Eating the right foods has also been shown to have a positive impact in boosting deep sleep, which I will discuss further in Chapter 6.

Deep sleep and memory

As well as giving your brain a good spring clean, deep sleep is when your brain sorts out your memories and shifts the useful ones into deep storage.

During an average waking day, an awful lot happens to you. You listen to the news, read a book, go to work, talk with friends, go on social media, listen to music. In other words, you load your brain with a myriad of potential memories. Some are useful, but others can be happily discarded. It is while you are asleep (particularly in deep sleep) that your brain decides which memories it wants to keep and which to discard.

It's a bit like sorting out photos and videos on your phone. Storing images requires a lot of memory, so when your phone starts to get full, you have to edit them. Removing dud videos and photos leaves space for new ones.

Even compared to a modern computer, your brain can store an extraordinary amount of data; a recent estimate puts its storage capacity at around 1000 terabytes, which is a billion megabytes. A computer with that capacity could store around 2 billion books or 500,000 films.

Yet while you have an awesome capacity to remember things, you don't want to store more junk up top than necessary. So, during the night, the memories that are considered important are shifted from the hippocampus (the short-term storage area of the brain) to the safety of the prefrontal cortex (the long-term storage area of the brain – think of it as your hard drive). The memories left behind in short-term storage are gradually deleted. That's why, if you are a student, getting a good night's sleep before an exam is so important. Staying up late and cramming is self-defeating because all those last-minute facts being madly forced in will soon be gone. You might think: 'I'll cut back on sleep during the week and then make up for it at the weekend.' Unfortunately, it doesn't work like that, because memories need to be consolidated within 24 hours of being formed.

A dramatic fall in the amount of deep sleep we typically get as we age may also explain why our ability to remember things gets worse as we get older.

In a recent study, researchers from the University of California, Berkeley,[2] asked 18 healthy young adults (mostly in their twenties) and 15 healthy older adults (who were mostly in their seventies) to come into the sleep lab to take part in a memory test. Before going to bed, they were asked to memorise pairs of words, and were tested to see how well they did.

They were then attached to an EEG machine, which measured their brainwave activity while they slept. The next morning, they were tested again to see how many of the word pairs they could recall.

The researchers found that the older participants got 75% less deep sleep than the younger participants, and their ability to remember word pairs was 55% worse.

Brain scans also showed that, overnight, the youngsters were much more efficient when it came to shifting memories from the short-term storage of the hippocampus to the long-term storage of the prefrontal cortex.

One encouraging finding was that applying 'transcranial direct current stimulation' – a small electric buzz to the surface of the brain – enhanced deep sleep in the older participants and improved their ability to do well in the memory test. Even so, as you'll discover in Chapter 7, there are easier ways to enhance deep sleep than giving your brain electric shocks.

REM sleep and emotions

As we've seen, deep sleep is vital for cleaning out our brains and sorting our memories. REM sleep, which occurs later in the night, is also important for tidying and organising our memories; but it has the additional role of helping resolve our emotional issues.

Although we dream at other points in the night, REM sleep is when we have our most vivid dreams, and it is these dreams that help us process and deal with bad memories and experiences. All of which helps explain another very odd finding: during REM sleep most of our muscles are paralysed. This is probably so that, while in the grips of an intense, dramatic dream, we don't thrash around and hurt ourselves. We do go on breathing, taking short, shallow breaths, but apart from that, the only part of us that is obviously moving is our eyes.

If you look at someone in REM sleep, you will see that, underneath their eyelids, their eyes are flicking madly to and fro. No one knows why this happens, but one theory is that it reflects the sort of eye movements you might make while watching a film. Dreams have been called the cinema of the mind, so perhaps the eye movements are simply a sign that you are following the action.

So how does REM sleep help us process our emotions? Well, it is all to do with the amygdalae, the two almond-shaped groups of cells located deep in the brain that play a key part in regulating emotions. Let's first look at how they work while we are awake.

I am mildly claustrophobic and, when I am in a confined space, I start to feel a sense of rising panic. That is because my amygdalae have triggered the release of 'fight or flight' hormones, such as adrenaline, and this in turn makes my heart rate, blood pressure and breathing shoot up. I feel nervous, sweaty and sometimes nauseous. There is a part of me that knows nothing bad is going to happen, but most of me just wants to escape from the situation.

Since the release of 'fight or flight' hormones plays such a big part in generating fear responses, I was fascinated to discover that REM sleep is the one time of day or night when links to these stress-inducing chemicals in the brain are switched off. This means that, while the dreams we have during REM sleep can be scary and disturbing, they are nothing like as bad as they would be if you were having them while you were awake.

Looked at this way, dreaming during REM sleep is a form of psychotherapy, where you revisit unpleasant memories and events but remain calm. This allows you to process your emotions and defuse them.

The Spider dream

While writing this book, I asked lots of people about their sleep and their dreams. The following story, which someone told me, is a great example of a therapeutic dream: 'When I was young I had a fear of spiders; it wasn't terrible but I had to leave the room if I saw one. Then one night I had a dream in which I was sitting on a chair in a dark room. From the chair I could see a door. There was a light under the door and I noticed that small spiders were crawling through the gap under the door. Slowly the gap under the door got bigger and bigger and as it did larger and larger spiders started coming through. For some reason I wasn't scared, I was just curious to see how big they would get. Then I woke up. The oddest thing is that after I had that dream, I wasn't scared of spiders any more. In fact the next time I saw one I was able to pick it up without shrieking.'

Sleep your way to the top

One other great thing about REM sleep is that it makes us more creative. It seems that the age-old advice about 'sleeping on a problem' is spot on: research has shown that a good night's sleep, particularly one that is rich in REM, increases our ability to come up with novel solutions to problems.

When I am struggling with a problem, I often write it down in a notebook, put it aside and then go back to it the next morning. I find it really helps. Decisions made late at night, or after a bad night's sleep, are often the ones we regret.

There are lots of lovely stories about people who have had their eureka moments while they slept.

- The writer Mary Godwin (later Mary Shelley) came up with the idea of Frankenstein after having a dream about a scientist who created life and was horrified by what he had done.
- Paul McCartney says the tune for 'Yesterday' came to him while he was asleep.
- Even more impressively, Keith Richards says he not only dreamed the opening lines to what would become one of the Rolling Stones' greatest hits, but played the song in his sleep. The story goes that he often kept a guitar and tape recorder by his bed, and one morning in May 1965, while on tour in Florida, he woke to find that the recorder had been running during the night. When he played it back, he heard himself playing the opening verse to 'Satisfaction'.
- Since REM sleep is all about excitable neuron activity in the brain, it is appropriate that the scientist Otto Loewi, who first showed us how nerves communicate, made his remarkable breakthrough thanks to a dream. In the spring of 1920, Dr Loewi was a frustrated man. He was convinced that nerve messages were transmitted using chemical signals, but he had spent 17 years trying to prove this and failed. Then, during the night of Easter Sunday 1920, he had a dream. He woke and jotted down a few notes on a slip of paper, before falling asleep again. When he woke up the next morning, he remembered he had written down something important, but when he picked up the paper he couldn't read his

own handwriting. Nor could he remember anything about the dream. Fortunately, the next night he had the same dream. This time he woke up properly and wrote the whole thing down. In the dream he was performing an experiment on frogs that would allow him to test his theory. As he later wrote: 'I got up immediately, went to the laboratory, and performed a simple experiment on a frog heart according to the nocturnal design.' The experiment worked and later won him the Nobel Prize in Medicine.

Things that go wrong if you don't get a decent night's sleep

WHY LACK OF SLEEP MAKES YOU FAT

A bad night's sleep not only affects your brain, but also messes with your body, including its ability to control your blood sugar levels. In the long run, this can lead to obesity and diabetes.

A few years ago, to see what impact even a couple of nights of reduced sleep can have, I took part in an experiment with Dr Eleanor Scott, who works at the University of Leeds. We recruited a group of healthy volunteers and fitted them with activity monitors and continuous glucose monitors – devices that are strapped to the arm to measure blood sugar levels. In this way, we were able to constantly monitor what was happening to their blood sugar levels without having to prick their fingers repeatedly.

First, we asked our volunteers to sleep normally for two nights (so we had a baseline to work from), then go to bed three hours later than normal for two nights. I felt I couldn't ask our volunteers to do this experiment unless I was ready to do it myself. I was also curious to see what effects it would have on my blood sugar levels. Back in 2012, I had discovered that I had type 2 diabetes, which I managed to get rid of by putting myself on the 5:2 diet and losing 20lb (9kg). Would a couple of nights' bad sleep set me back, even now?

After two nights of severe sleep deprivation, I went back up to Leeds, where I met up with Dr Scott and the other volunteers. Everyone complained about having the munchies.

As one of them put it: 'I wanted lots of biscuits and I didn't just have one. I'd go for 10 custard creams.'

'Is that unusual?' I asked him.

'Well, it's certainly unusual for breakfast!'

All of us, whether we had feasted on biscuits or managed to stick to our normal diet, saw marked increases in our blood sugar levels when we were badly sleep deprived, to the point where some of us (myself included), who had normal levels at the start of the experiment, now had those you would expect to see in a type 2 diabetic. Our blood sugars returned to normal after a good night's sleep.

As Dr Scott pointed out, there is now a lot of evidence that people who sleep badly most nights are far more likely to become overweight or obese and develop type 2 diabetes than those who sleep really well. So why does this happen? 'We know that when you are sleep deprived,' Dr Scott said, 'this alters your appetite hormones, making you more likely to feel hungry and less likely to feel full. We also know that when people are sleep deprived, they often crave sweet foods, which could explain the custard cream cravings. Also, if you're awake when you're not meant to be, you produce more of the stress hormone cortisol, and that can influence your glucose level as well the next day.'

Ours was quite a small experiment, but a recent meta-analysis, carried out by researchers at King's College London,[3] found that sleep-deprived people consume, on average, an extra 385 calories per day, which is equivalent to a large slice of cake.

It's not just that your blood sugar levels soar and your hunger hormones go into overdrive when you're tired; the areas of your brain associated with reward also become more active. In other words, you become much more motivated than normal to seek out unhealthy foods such as crisps and chocolate.

Another study[4] showed that children are affected in a similar way. Researchers took a group of children aged between three and four years, all regular afternoon nappers, and not only deprived them of their afternoon nap but also kept them up for about two hours past their normal bedtime. The following day, the children ate 21% more calories than usual, including 25% more sugary snacks. They were then allowed to sleep as much as they wanted. The next day, they still consumed 14% more calories than they had before being deprived of sleep.

THE VICIOUS CIRCLE

Lack of sleep makes you fatter, but piling on extra fat (particularly around the gut and neck) also means you sleep worse. It is a vicious circle. When I was an overweight diabetic, I slept badly, at least in part because I snored so much. Being overweight also greatly increases your risk of having sleep apnoea, a disorder that causes you to stop breathing hundreds of times a night. This will make you really tired and hungry and it is terrible for the brain.

A Swedish study[5] showed just how disruptive being overweight is when it comes to sleep. For the study, the researchers recruited 400 women with an average age of 50 from the town of Uppsala. Half the women were overweight and had 'central obesity', meaning their waists measured more than 88cm (35in). The other half were slimmer, with a Body Mass Index (BMI) in the normal range. After being weighed and having their waists measured, the women were led away to the sleeping area, where the team hooked them up to sleep recorders. The women were then allowed to sleep for as long as they wanted. The differences in sleep quality and quantity were striking. The women with less belly fat slept, on average, 25 minutes more per night. They also got 20% more brain-restoring deep sleep and 22% more emotionally calming REM sleep.

METABOLIC SYNDROME

Lack of sleep also contributes to metabolic syndrome, which is the medical term for a cluster of conditions that includes too much body fat around the waist, raised blood pressure, blood sugar and cholesterol, which in turn lead to an increased risk of type 2 diabetes, stroke and heart disease. Metabolic syndrome, also known as Syndrome X, affects around 1 in 4 adults in the UK (and 1 in 3 Australians) and has a major impact on future health, not only because it encourages further build-up of fat, particularly around your gut (visceral fat), but because it leads to increased insulin resistance. In other words, your body has to pump out ever increasing amounts of insulin to bring your blood sugars back to normal.

LOW MOOD

Anyone who has been sleep deprived knows that it leads to anger and irritability, while at the same time sucking the joy out of life. If you are feeling anxious and depressed this will, in turn, affect how well you sleep. Being agitated keeps your body and brain aroused, just when you want them to wind down. More on how to combat this in Chapter 5.

SEX DRIVE

As well as making you feel simply 'too tired for sex', being sleep deprived suppresses the production of the two main sex hormones, oestrogen and testosterone. This, in turn, has a devastating effect on sexual desire.

The good news is that getting more sleep should improve your sex drive. A two-week study[6] of 171 American women found that an extra hour of sleep increased the chance that they would want to have sex the following night by 14%.

But does it work the other way round? Will having more sex improve your sleep? In theory it should, as regular sex boosts levels of the hormone oxytocin (also known as the 'love hormone' because it helps human bonding) while reducing levels of stress hormones like cortisol. But it seems to be a more effective sleep aid if you are male than if you are female.

In a recent survey[7] carried out by researchers from Central Queensland University, 68% of the male respondents said that having sex improved the quality of their sleep, compared to 59% of female respondents. Another enlightening finding was that 11% of women said that sex with their partner made their sleep worse, compared with just 4% of men.

How lack of sleep impacts on your health

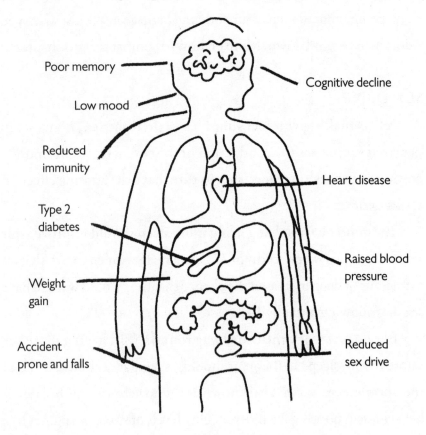

The researchers thought this gender difference was probably because the men were more likely to report having had an orgasm during sex than the women. They added that, 'while orgasms with a partner appear to have the most benefit in terms of sleep outcomes, orgasms achieved through self-stimulation can also aid sleep quality'. They called for further research ...

Keeping track of your sleep

It's all very well being told that getting enough sleep is vital for your brain, your waist and your sex life, but how do you track how much you are getting? Most people don't have access to a sleep lab.

Without an EEG machine you won't get a very accurate picture of your sleep, but some of the more modern sleep trackers, which also measure your heart rate, do a reasonable job. I spent some time looking into trackers and in the end I went for the Fitbit Alta HR Activity Tracker with Heart Rate Monitor.

The Fitbit Alta HR has been the subject of proper clinical trials, including a recent study[8] where researchers from Monash University in Australia compared the accuracy of the tracker with the data collected from 49 people linked to machines in a sleep lab. The researchers concluded that the watch was pretty good at telling when people were in deep sleep and REM sleep, but tended to overestimate how much sleep people got because it was not great at detecting when people were awake but not moving.

And if you are the anxious sort, then be warned that being told by your machine that you're not getting enough of the right sort of sleep can induce further anxiety.

When my device told me I was getting less deep sleep than I needed, I became obsessed with the need for more – and stayed awake worrying about it. There is even a condition known as orthosomnia, which describes an unhealthy obsession with getting the right amount of 'healthy' sleep each night.

The term was coined a few years ago by sleep researchers at North-western University in the US who had noticed that they were seeing lots of patients whose quest for a perfect night's rest had led, ironically, to sleep problems.

They wrote that on one occasion they had carried out tests on a 27-year-old woman who was complaining of poor sleep. The tests showed that she had slept well. Her response was: 'Then why does my fitness tracker say I slept poorly?'

So, if you use these devices to track your sleep, take the results with a pinch of salt; I do think it is worth buying one, as that will make it much easier to calculate and track your sleep efficiency. That said, I strongly recommend that you keep a sleep diary as well.

A SLEEP DIARY

I wore the tracker for several months, while keeping a detailed sleep diary, and the tracker did seem to reflect how much I had slept and how well I had slept. I have included a copy of a daily page from a sleep diary in Chapter 7, and you can download more copies at www.fast-asleep. com/sleep-diary. If you are curious about your sleep, and certainly if you suffer from any form of insomnia, then keeping a sleep diary is an absolute must. I will go into the whys and wherefores later.

SLEEP EFFICIENCY

As I mentioned a moment ago, one of the other things that a sleep tracker will allow you to do is calculate your sleep efficiency, which is a core part of the 4-Week Sleep Plan; it is a measure of the amount of time you spend in bed actually asleep.

Let me illustrate with my own example.

I try to be in bed by 11pm and get up at 7am most days of the week, including weekends. Routine is hugely important if you want to sleep well, and I value my sleep.

My sleep tracker told me that over the course of a month I was in bed for an average of 7 hours and 50 minutes a night, but I was only asleep for 6 hours and 40 minutes. The rest of the time I was trying to sleep, roaming the house or reading.

If you translate that into minutes you can calculate my sleep efficiency:

$$(6 \times 60) + 40/(7 \times 60) + 50 = 400/470 = 85\%$$

Eighty-five per cent is actually pretty good. In fact, anything between 85% and 90% is excellent, and very few people have a sleep efficiency that is over 90%. An insomniac will probably spend around 70% of the night asleep.

And what about the different stages of sleep? According to my tracker, of the 6 hours and 40 minutes that I was asleep, I was in deep sleep for 17% and in REM for 18% of the time. The rest of the time I was in light sleep.

Which isn't bad. According to a Fitbit study,[9] the average user lies awake for 55 minutes every night and sleeps for around 6 hours and 33 minutes. They are in deep sleep for 15% and in REM for about 20%.

Again, according to Fitbit, the older you are the less sleep you tend to get, down from 6 hours and 58 minutes for young adults, to 6 hours and 33 minutes for people aged 52 and older. The big drop was in the amount of deep sleep people got as they aged, down from 71 minutes a night to just 50 minutes for the over 50s.

In the Fitbit study, the women got slightly more sleep than the men, by about 25 minutes a night, and this is reflected in other studies of American adults.

It seems that women put a higher priority on sleep, perhaps because they are better at recognising the health benefits. There is also evidence that women are more vulnerable to the impact of sleep deprivation.

Summary

- There are three distinct states of sleep: light sleep, deep sleep and REM sleep.
- During the night we sleep in roughly 90-minute cycles, with most deep sleep happening in the early part of the night, and most REM sleep happening later on.
- Around half the night is spent in light sleep.
- Deep sleep is when your brain gets cleaned and your memories get sorted.
- REM sleep is when you have vivid dreams that help you process your emotions.
- Not getting enough sleep increases your risk of obesity, type 2 diabetes, dementia, raised blood pressure and low mood. It also reduces your sex drive.
- The really important thing is not how long you spend in bed but how long you spend in bed ASLEEP. Being able to estimate your sleep efficiency is key to doing the 4-Week Sleep Plan.

2. What puts us to sleep

The urge to sleep begins early in the day, from the moment that you first wake up and get out of bed. Shortly before you wake, your body releases a surge of hormones, including the stress hormone cortisol, which prepares you for the day. But waking also triggers the release of a chemical in the brain called adenosine. Adenosine binds to receptors in your brain, slowing down brain activity. This suppression of brain cell activity is what causes the feeling of drowsiness.

The longer you are awake, the higher your adenosine levels rise. The higher the adenosine levels, the sleepier you get. Then, when you finally go to bed and sleep, the adenosine is broken up and disposed of.

If you are feeling sleepy and want to stay awake, you can, temporarily, block the effects of adenosine by consuming the world's most popular psychoactive drug, caffeine. Caffeine binds to sleep-inducing receptors in your brain that would otherwise be occupied by adenosine – that's why it wakes you up.

As you may have noticed, caffeine has very different effects on different people. There are some people, like my wife, who are really sensitive to caffeine. She only needs one cup to wake her up. Caffeine also hangs around in her system for much longer than it does in mine.

The reason you have to keep topping up your caffeine is that it is constantly being broken down by your liver. The average half-life of caffeine is around five hours, which means that, if you have a cup of coffee at 6pm, half is still running around your system at 11pm and a quarter is still there at 4am.

If you are sensitive to caffeine, you will still be feeling the effects of an afternoon cup of coffee in the middle of the night, lying awake and wondering why you can't sleep.

But quoting average figures is misleading because some people break down caffeine much faster than others. The 'average' half-life of caffeine may be five hours, but the range is actually 1.5 hours to nine hours.

If you are someone whose body breaks down caffeine especially slowly, you will still be feeling the effects of your morning cup of tea or coffee in the middle of the night. But, if you are naturally able to break down caffeine rapidly, then you can drink coffee in the evening without it disturbing your sleep.

Various things affect the half-life of caffeine in your body, including your gender, age, weight and any medication you are on. Taking the oral contraceptive pill will dramatically slow your liver's ability to break it down.

The biggest factor, however, is your personal genetics. If you are interested, you can get yourself genetically tested by companies like 23andme.com. You order a test online, and a few days later they send you a plastic tube. You spit in the tube and send it back. A few weeks later, you log in and see what they have found.

I did this a few years ago and I found the results fascinating. According to 23andme, their test suggests that I am unlikely to have developed a bald spot (true) or get dandruff (true) but I can probably smell the asparagus odour in my urine (also true). As for caffeine, it turns out that I am more sensitive than most and I would be well advised to drink less of the stuff. These days, I have two to three cups of coffee during the morning and rarely drink any after midday.

DON'T DRINK COFFEE FOR AN HOUR AFTER GETTING UP

And it is also best to avoid drinking coffee within an hour of getting up in the morning, or at least wait until you are having breakfast, particularly if you have had disrupted sleep. I got this bit of advice from Dr James Betts, who is Professor of Metabolic Physiology at the University of Bath. He told me that his research has shown that drinking coffee straight after a poor night's sleep can lead to a 50% bigger surge in your blood sugar levels when you have breakfast than if you delay the coffee until after eating.

Even if you have slept well, you will still experience a rise in your cortisol levels (this is known as CAR, or cortisol arousal response), which starts a couple of hours before you wake and peaks an hour or so after you get up.

So it is best to hit your body with caffeine when your cortisol levels are falling, not while they are still high. If you drink coffee when cortisol levels are high, you will soon develop tolerance to it; in other words, you will find you need to drink more of it to get the same kick. For both these reasons Professor Betts recommends delaying that first coffee until breakfast or later to minimise its negative effects on your blood sugar level.

Your internal clocks

As well as the build-up of adenosine, the other major driver of sleep is your circadian clock. Deep in your brain there is a small group of cells called the suprachiasmatic nucleus (SCN). If I were to drill a hole between your eyebrows and carry on drilling into your brain until I hit the hypothalamus, and if I were then to stick an electrode down that hole, you would actually be able to hear the clock tick.

Oddly enough, your circadian clock doesn't follow a day that is exactly 24 hours long. Some people's clock runs fast, others' runs slow. If you have a fast clock then that means you are a lark – you like to get up early. If you have a slow clock then you are an owl, someone who likes to stay up late. The reason you don't go completely out of whack is that your internal clock is reset every day by light.

Rays of light from the sun hit receptors in the back of your eyes that have nothing to do with vision but instead are linked to the SCN. The SCN then sends out signals to other parts of your body, including your guts, letting them know that a new day has begun and it is time to get moving. It's a bit like shouting at the kids, 'Wake up, breakfast will be on the table in 20 minutes.'

Similarly, just as we like to have a warm house when we get up, the SCN raises your core body temperature before you wake, so you are ready to get going. It will also, in the early hours of the morning, switch off the production of melatonin – a hormone connected to your brain clock that is released when it gets dark to help tip you into sleep (more on that later) – and switch on the release of the stress hormone cortisol.

What makes things a bit more complicated is the fact that each of our organs has its own clock, which is linked to the main clock but not necessarily driven by it. The clock in your liver, for example, is not reset by light but by when you eat. This is important, because when your biological clocks get out of sync with the outside world, and with each other, you are in trouble. Not only will you struggle to sleep, but you will get hungry, have problems controlling your blood sugar levels, feel run down and tired, and find it hard to concentrate. It's called 'social jet lag', because just like the jet lag you experience after travelling across multiple time zones, it leaves you feeling terrible.

Fortunately, you can retune your clocks and get your body back into sync with some relatively straightforward tweaks. These involve making sure you eat the right food, at the right time, and that you get exposure to strong enough light, again at the right time. That is what this book will help you do. Fix the clocks. Fast.

Larks and owls

Some people leap out of bed in the morning, raring to go. Others need an alarm clock – preferably two – to get them off to work on time.

My wife will quite happily stay up working until the small hours, while I prefer to head for bed soon after 10pm. I'm a lark; Clare is an owl. I'm itching to leave a party by 11pm; she is just warming up. We have different chronotypes and there is good evidence that this is not just personal preference but has roots in our genes.

For a bit of insight into what mine say about my sleeping patterns, I dropped in on Dr Simon Archer, who is Professor of Molecular Biology of Sleep at the University of Surrey. Among other things, Simon has conducted studies looking at links between an individual's genetic markers and how vulnerable they are to sleep loss.

I had sent him the raw data from my 23andme gene test and he had taken a close look. What did his team make of it?

'Well,' he said, 'the first thing that stood out is you have three genetic markers that would predict you are a morning-type person.' He then added, 'We also found a marker for increased risk of insomnia and a marker which is associated with poor sleep efficiency in people who are exposed to high levels of work-related stress.

'From what I've seen, I would predict that you often have disrupted, fragmented sleep during the night and that you need more sleep than most.'

All of which is true. I get really grumpy and sleep badly when I am stressed.

So my genes test confirmed what I had long suspected: that I am one of those people whose circadian clock is a little fast, meaning that I like to get up early and go to bed early.

Can you tell if you are a lark or an owl without doing a genetic test? Try answering the following seven questions with a straightforward 'yes' or 'no'.

1. Do you wake up bright and cheerful, without an alarm clock, by 7am?
2. If you go to bed at 10pm, do you swiftly fall asleep?
3. Do you always try to head to bed before midnight, even if you are on holiday?
4. Or do you have trouble falling asleep before midnight?
5. Do you need an alarm clock to drag you out of bed in the morning?
6. Do you find you don't need to eat until later in the day and are happy with just a coffee?
7. Given the chance, would you sleep in till 11am or later?

If you answered 'yes' to the first three questions and 'no' to the last four, you have strong larkish tendencies. If it was the other way around, you are more owlish.

Why larks turn into owls and back again

When it comes to your chronotype, it is not just about your genes. Both your age and gender also play a role.

A big study of 25,000 people of all ages who were asked to fill in a

ChronoType Questionnaire[10] found that while most children are larks (early chronotypes), they become progressively more owlish through the teenage years, hitting maximum 'owlishness' at around the age of 20. They try to sneak their phones up to their bedrooms, stay up late chatting to their friends on social media and are hard to rouse in the morning. They grunt at breakfast, refuse your healthy offerings and instead buy junk food and energy drinks on the way to school to wake themselves up.

Yes, this behaviour is really annoying but, to some extent, it's not their fault. When puberty comes along, it shifts the internal clock to a later setting, by an average of one to two hours. So an angelic child who was once quite happy to go to bed by 9.30pm and get up at 7am (getting the necessary 10 hours in bed) is now a stroppy teenager who resents being sent to bed at all and resents even more getting up at 7am, after having managed less than seven hours' sleep. And there are clear gender differences. Girls, who tend to hit puberty earlier than boys, also start turning owlish earlier, reaching 'maximum owl' at the age of 19, before slowly becoming more larkish. Boys, on the other hand, have a body clock that tends to get them to bed later and later, until they hit the age of 21 and have to fit into the adult world. None the less, they tend to remain more owlish than women until they hit their fifties, when gender differences disappear.

This is a real pain for both parents and offspring, because it causes a lot of conflict, but that may actually be what Nature intended. When kids are young, it is vital that their parents nurture and look after them. But as they grow older, they need to start to assert their own identity, to prepare for life outside the parental home, where they will have to fend for themselves, just as our ancestors did when they left the safety of the tribe. Staying up late, with other teenagers, while the parents are all asleep, may be Nature's way of bonding the next generation together.

The trouble is, the modern world doesn't allow a lie-in. If you are a teenager, you may have an internal clock telling you to stay up late and get up late, but you also have parents who are shouting at you that it is time to get dressed and go to school. The result is that most teenagers burn the candle at both ends and fewer than 25% get the recommended nine to ten hours during school time. The obvious solution would be to start the school day later, and lots of schools have tried this. In 2016, the US city of Seattle announced that most of its middle school and all its high schools would start an hour later – putting arrival time back from 7.50am to 8.45am. Parents were not keen and all the extracurricular schedules had to be changed, so there was a lot of grumbling from the staff. But was it worth it?

Well, researchers asked 170 students from two of the schools who were about to make the change to wear activity monitors to track their sleep. They found that putting school time back by almost an hour did indeed have a big effect on the amount these students slept. It went up from an average of six hours and 50 minutes, before the change, to seven hours and 24 minutes afterwards, an added 34 minutes of sleep each night. Academic performance and school attendance also improved impressively, in line with getting more sleep.

Another study,[11] this time in Fairfax, Virginia, showed that delaying the start of the school day can cut car accidents. They found that students aged between 16 and 18 who drove themselves to school were nearly 9% less likely to have a crash if they went to a school where the day started later.

Turning an owl into a lark

Being a night owl leads to fights with your parents when you are a teenager and can be extremely inconvenient as you get older.

I recently met a night owl called Marie, who works full time and has two young children aged three and five. She has been a night owl since her teens and she told me that she would, given half a chance, stay up until two or three in the morning and wake up at around 11am.

Because she has young children she can't sleep in, and anyway, she has a job that involves a 9am start. So she goes to bed around 11pm most nights, but then lies there awake until 2am or later.

She is rudely awoken by her alarm clock at 7am, or by her children clamouring to be let into the bedroom. Her husband, who is also something of an owl, is able to function perfectly fine on five or six hours' sleep a night. But Marie can't. She told me that she wakes up most mornings feeling absolutely shattered.

She has tried all the obvious things such as exercise and not lying in at weekends, but nothing works, except for sleeping pills, and that is not a road she wants to go down in the long term.

The good news for people like Marie is that it is possible, in just three weeks, to turn yourself from an owl into a lark, and without drugs.

You do it by resetting your internal clocks. And you do that by controlling exposure to light and the timing of your meals.

To show it can be done, researchers from Monash University in Australia recruited 22 owls, men and women who normally go to bed around 2.30am and wake up at 10am.[12]

For three weeks they were asked to follow nine simple rules. These were:

1. To wake up at least two hours earlier than normal, which for this group meant getting up by 8am.
2. To get outside and expose themselves to plenty of outdoor light in the mornings.
3. To have breakfast as soon as convenient.
4. To only exercise in the morning.
5. To have lunch at the same time every day.
6. To avoid all caffeine after 4pm.
7. To avoid having a nap after 4pm.
8. To avoid bright lights during the evening and to head to bed a couple of hours earlier than normal – i.e. by about midnight.
9. To stick to this regime every day of the week, including weekends.

After three weeks, the owls had successfully shifted their body clocks forward by an impressive two hours. Not only were they going to sleep earlier, but tests showed that their levels of melatonin, the sleep-inducing hormone, were peaking two hours earlier.

Having shifted their body clocks they felt far less sleepy during the day and reported feeling happier with their lives in general. Their depression and stress scores improved, as well as their performance in cognitive tests. They even got physically stronger.

I'm pleased to say that Marie followed this advice and now finds going to sleep and getting up at a normal time very much easier.

Camping, anyone?

An even quicker way to convert yourself from an owl to a lark could be to go camping. A few years ago, Dr Kenneth Wright of the University of Boulder in Colorado sent eight people (six men and two women) on a camping trip to the Rocky Mountains.[13] He gave them wrist monitors to record how much light they were being exposed to, and activity monitors to measure how much sleep they were getting. During the week that they were away camping, they were not allowed torches or mobile phones, and the only light they saw at night was from candles or the campfire.

Their monitors showed that over the course of the week they were exposed to four times their normal levels of light. This had a big effect on their sleeping patterns.

Before they went camping, their average bedtime was 12.30am; by the time they got home it was more like 11pm. Their sleep was now much more in sync with sunrise and sunset.

When he tested their blood in the lab, Dr Wright found that the participants' bodies had started to release melatonin two hours earlier than they had before the trip. He had turned owls into larks in just one week. Who knows, it might even work on teenagers.

3. What keeps us awake

My idea of a great night's sleep is to go to bed around 11pm, fall asleep within a few minutes and then wake up, refreshed, at about 7am, without the need for an alarm clock. That would be lovely. It is what used to happen. It hardly ever happens now.

I have no problem getting to bed and falling asleep, but I almost always wake up in the middle of the night, and sometimes find it hard to get back to sleep. In this respect, I am a classic insomniac.

There are other types of insomnia: not being able to get to sleep is quite common, as is waking up early in the morning. But the most common form is waking in the middle of the night, particularly as we get older. This is partly because our sleep gets lighter as we age, but also because of things like having a full bladder and feeling the need to go to the toilet.

I used to get quite worked up about this. I resented the fact that no matter how tired I was, I'd wake up four and a half hours after going to sleep (normally around 3.30am). I would go to the loo, get back into bed and then just lie there, for what felt like hours, worrying about not being able to get back to sleep, and worrying about how tired I would feel in the morning. Finally, I'd drift off, only to be dragged awake again by the alarm clock at 7am.

Then, a few years ago, while researching a documentary about life in Victorian slums, I interviewed Roger Ekirch, a professor of history at Virginia Tech in the US. He told me that my pattern – falling asleep, waking for a while, then falling asleep again – was how many people slept in pre-industrial times. Apparently, people would go to bed around 9pm, sleep for about five hours, then get up at about 2am. They would do household chores, visit friends or 'enjoy a bit of intimacy', before heading to bed again for a 'second sleep'. Professor Ekirch believes that the pressures of the industrial age and the arrival of electric lights changed all that; sleeping continuously became the new normal. And, as the practice of sleeping continuously became more widespread, the idea of a 'first' and 'second' sleep faded from public consciousness. Even napping, which can be hugely beneficial (see page 138) and which used to be very common in hot countries, has largely been abandoned.

To support his claims that biphasic sleeping (sleeping in two blocks) has deep roots, Professor Ekirch pointed me towards research done by Dr Thomas Wehr, a psychiatrist at the National Institute of Mental Health.[14]

In the early 1990s, Dr Wehr conducted an experiment in which he persuaded a group of healthy volunteers to spend a month in a lab, where it was pitch black for 14 hours of the day.

By the end of the experiment, the volunteers were sleeping an average of eight hours a night, but not in one block. Instead, they slept for three to five hours, woke for an hour or two and then fell back asleep for a second block of three to five hours.

Carol Worthman, an anthropologist at Emory University in Atlanta, thinks there may be something in Professor Ekirch's claims. She has studied the sleep patterns of hunter-gatherers who follow a pre-industrial way of life. She says that interrupted or polyphasic sleep is quite normal among them. In many of the tribes she has studied, she has found around one in four people are up and active at any given point in the night. She thinks that there may be an evolutionary advantage to this, because when our remote ancestors lived out in the open it would have been important that at least some of the tribe were awake, alert and looking out for predators.

If, like me, you often find yourself awake in the middle of the night, you can console yourself with the thought that humans have probably been doing this for thousands of years. Buoyed by these discoveries, I decided that rather than fight my 'old-fashioned' sleeping patterns, I'd work with them. So these days I accept that I will probably wake at about 3am and plan accordingly. If I have an early start, then I aim to be in bed by 10.30pm. This gives me a roughly four-and-a-half-hour 'first sleep'.

When I wake around 3am, rather than lie there fretting, I get up and go to another room, where I listen to music, meditate or read a really boring book. I keep a special collection of books for this purpose. When I start to feel sleepy, which is normally after around 40 minutes, I go back to bed for three or so hours of 'second' sleep.

Between my first and second sleep, I take care to avoid doing anything exciting or stimulating. If you are awake in the night your goal should be to bore your brain into going back to sleep.

Since I have, slightly reluctantly, accepted that I am unlikely to return to sleeping for a whole night without a break, I've felt more rested, less stressed and much less likely to nod off during the day. Try it for yourself, and let me know how you get on.

Snoring

Along with having a full bladder, one of the main reasons why people sleep badly is that they or their partner snore. I come from a long line of snorers. My father used to snore really, really loudly, like someone sawing logs. It was loud enough to be heard on the other side of the house.

I also used to snore at an incredible volume; in fact, my wife said that when we lived in London, I snored so loudly that I drowned out the sound of the metal beer barrels being delivered to the pub opposite first thing in the morning.

Although the caricature of a snorer is a fat, middle-aged man, women also snore. A few years ago, British newspapers outed a grandmother of four as 'one of Britain's loudest snorers'. She was recorded snoring at a window-rattling 112 decibels, which meant her snoring was louder than the noise made by a low-flying jet. According to the papers, it was loud enough to drown out a 'diesel truck, farm tractor or speeding express train'. Apparently, her husband coped by sleeping in the spare room and burying his head in a pillow.

I don't know if this was her problem, but the main reason most people snore is that they are overweight. If you are a woman with a neck size over 16 inches (41cm), or a man with a neck size over 17 inches (43cm), you are almost certainly a snorer.

As we get older and fatter, we snore more. That's because our throat gets narrower, our throat muscles get weaker and our uvula, which is that finger-like bit of tissue that hangs down at the back of our throat, gets floppier. All these changes mean that when we breathe in, the air can't move freely through our nose and throat and into our lungs. Instead, the incoming air makes the surrounding tissues vibrate, which produces that horrendous snoring noise.

Snoring and sleep apnoea

As well as being annoying, snoring can be a sign of Obstructive Sleep Apnoea (OSA), which is much more worrying. OSA occurs when muscles at the back of the throat relax and temporarily restrict or block airflow as you sleep, which leads to falling blood oxygen levels. This, combined with an increase in blood pressure, puts you at increased risk of having a heart attack.

It can kill you. The actress Carrie Fisher, famous as Princess Leia in Star Wars, died from a heart attack at the age of 60 while on a plane. The coroner said that the main contributory factors were untreated sleep apnoea and a build-up of fatty tissue on the walls of her arteries.

An awful lot of people with sleep apnoea go untreated because they think it is just snoring and that snoring is harmless.

A couple of years ago I was on a train when an overweight middle-aged man called George introduced himself. He knew I wrote diet books but was keen to point out that he didn't believe in them and he certainly didn't need to diet.

I asked George if he had any trouble sleeping, and he admitted that he felt tired all the time. He also said he snored loudly, particularly after a few drinks, and that his wife had told him that there were times during the night when he stopped breathing.

He said he wasn't worried by this, but I was, particularly when he told me that he was a long-distance lorry driver and kept himself awake with energy drinks. I suggested that he get his wife to stay up for an hour or two to count how many times he stopped breathing. 'Stopping breathing' means not breathing for 10 seconds or longer. Other things to look out for in someone with sleep apnoea are regular gasping, snorting or choking noises, hypersomnia (excessive daytime sleepiness) and lack of interest in sex.

There are apps you can download, like Snore Control and SnoreLab which warn you that you might have sleep apnoea. Once you have downloaded one of these apps you just leave your smart phone by your bed. The app can, apparently, detect when you are snoring loudly; if you wake up gasping for air, or if you wake up making choking sounds.

If the app tells you there is something wrong, or if you are waking up a lot in the night and your partner says that you are making gasping, snoring or choking noises, then do see your doctor.

Other warning signs are waking up with a headache, feeling very tired during the day and finding it hard to concentrate. This is something that is really worth taking seriously because as well as leaving you feeling exhausted, it greatly increases your risk of heart attack and stroke. Sleep apnoea is strongly linked to insomnia, and if you have both (it is called COMISA), then the health risks are higher than having either condition alone.

OSA affects around one in four men and one in ten women. Unfortunately, it is particularly common in truck drivers, who tend to be overweight because they spend a lot of their working lives sitting on their bottoms eating junk. A recent study[15] of 905 Italian truck drivers found that around half suffered from a sleep-related breathing problem, making them dangerously prone to falling asleep at the wheel. I pointed out to George that having untreated OSA doubled his risk of sudden death. The fact that he was starving his brain of oxygen every night also increased his risk of Alzheimer's and dementia. He looked pensive.

I explained that the best way to cure his snoring and his sleep apnoea was to lose weight, fast. The reason I used to snore so loudly was because I used to have a 17-inch (43 cm) neck. When I put myself on the 5:2 diet, back in 2012, and lost 20lb (9kg), I also lost an inch (about 2.5 cm) of fat around my neck. I completely stopped snoring and our house was finally at peace.

I suggested to George that if he wanted to find out more about the advantages of rapid weight loss and how to do it safely, he should buy one of my books or visit thefast800.com. He said he would think about it. I like to think he followed through.

RAPID WEIGHT LOSS AND SLEEP APNOEA

Although slim people can develop OSA, it is far more common in people who store fat around the neck. As I told George, if you are overweight then rapid weight loss is the most effective way of curing snoring and OSA.

A study[16] carried out in Finland with overweight or obese patients diagnosed with mild OSA found that putting them on a rapid weight loss diet (800 calories a day for up to 12 weeks) cured more than half of them. They lost an average of 10.7kg, which dramatically improved their sleep as well as their hypertension, high cholesterol and raised blood sugar levels.

The greater the weight loss, the greater the improvement. Ninety per cent of those who lost more than 15kg were cured of OSA, but even if they lost and kept off just 3kg, their chance of a cure was still 38%.

If you have OSA, but are not overweight, or are not motivated to lose weight, you might benefit from a CPAP machine. CPAP stands for Continuous Positive Airway Pressure. It is a machine that sits beside your bed and pumps air into a mask covering your nose and sometimes your mouth while you are asleep. The idea is that the pressure of the air keeps your throat open so you don't stop breathing.

It can be a life saver. A woman I worked with discovered she had sleep apnoea and was prescribed a CPAP machine. Within a couple of weeks, she was transformed from a shattered wreck into a bundle of happy energy. 'I had no idea how awful I felt in the mornings until I stopped feeling awful,' she told me. Because she was feeling so much more energetic, she decided to follow my advice, did the Fast 800 diet, lost 15kg and was soon able to return her CPAP machine to the astonished sleep clinic.

You might expect the ferocity of snoring to gradually decrease as you lose weight. But this is very often not the case. There seems to be a critical tipping point. So don't be discouraged if, to start with, your snoring does not seem to be improving – get down to a healthy weight and it will get better. And remember that, even if it doesn't completely cure your snoring, you will get all those other health benefits of losing weight.

I mentioned earlier that getting a CPAP machine can be life changing, but they also have significant downsides. There is the cost, the inconvenience of having to carry it around with you when you are travelling and the fact that you have to wear a mask in bed every night. A bit of a passion killer, I would have thought. Around half of people who try out a CPAP machine are unable to tolerate it, for whatever reason.

Anti-snoring devices

In addition to CPAP machines, there are lots of anti-snoring devices you can buy, ranging from nasal strips that keep your nose open to 'mandibular advancement devices', which push your lower jaw and tongue forward, with the aim of opening up your airways.

The latter can really work wonders, but are best when specially fitted. If you get a referral to a sleep clinic, they may be able to offer you tailored advice; otherwise your best bet is to go online and see what your fellow snorers have bought and what they make of their purchases.

If you are really desperate, there is also uvulopalatopharyngo-plasty. This is an operation where a surgeon burns or cuts away tissue in your throat to try and clear the obstruction. This has risks, recovery is painful and it is not always effective, particularly if the main reason you have sleep apnoea is because you are overweight. It can make the condition worse.

Things that go bump in the night

As you may have gathered by now, things can get quite eventful in the Mosley household at night. Not only do I regularly roam around at 3am, but Clare sometimes gets up in the night, while remaining firmly asleep. Recently, she climbed over me and started looking through the clothes cupboard. When I asked her what she was doing, she said she was looking for a missing hamster that needed feeding. We haven't had hamsters for years. I persuaded her to go back to bed and she immediately fell fast asleep and had no memory of any of this the following morning. Clare has 'parasomnia', a common sleep disorder which includes a range of weird and wonderful things that can happen to people while they are asleep: sleepwalking, sleep talking, nightmares, sleep eating, sleep paralysis, sleep aggression and even sexsomnia (having sex when you are asleep), are all forms of parasomnia.

About 10% of the population have a parasomnia of some sort and though they can affect people at any age, they are more common in children, probably because children have immature brains.

Parasomnias also run in families, which could explain why two of my sons were sleepwalkers when they were young. We would often find them walking the corridors in the middle of the night. One of them managed to walk out of the front door, while fast asleep, and lock himself out. He spent half an hour banging on the door until one of us woke and let him in.

Sleepwalking can, of course, be extremely dangerous. When he was 10 years old, our oldest son managed to sleepwalk his way out of the first-floor bedroom window of a cottage where we were staying. He fell about 4.5 metres onto the flagstones below. We were unbelievably lucky that a neighbour, Russell, who happened to be wandering around outside at 3am, heard him cry out, investigated, found him unconscious and woke us. We wrapped his head in ice (I had recently made a documentary about how cooling can reduce the risk of brain injury) and he was rushed by ambulance to the local hospital, where an MRI scan revealed he had a fractured skull. To our huge relief he made a full recovery.

After that, we made sure that all the upstairs windows at home were secure. Fortunately, both boys stopped sleepwalking in their early teens.

Q&A

Should you try to wake someone who is sleepwalking, sleep eating or having some other parasomnia episode?
It is not a good idea to shake or shout at a person who is in the grip of parasomnia, as that may trigger an irritable, aggressive or even violent reaction. It is much better to mutter 'time for bed' and gently guide them back to their bedroom.

At what time of night does it happen?
It can happen at any time of the night, but it typically occurs when the person is coming out of deep sleep. One part of their brain is still in deep sleep, so they are unconscious, but other parts of their brain are awake enough that they can walk, talk, even drive. I met a woman who used to drive to work during the middle of the night, waking up in the company car park with no idea of how she had got there. She solved this problem by locking her car keys in the safe every evening.

Apparently, her unconscious mind could drive but couldn't remember the safe's combination.

Can you prevent parasomnia?
If your child or partner sleepwalks at the same time every night, you

could try gently waking them about half an hour before they would normally sleepwalk. By doing this, you disrupt their sleep cycle and in some cases that is enough to stop their parasomnia. You will need to do this every evening for at least a week to break the cycle.

If they are at serious risk of hurting themselves or someone else they should see their doctor – they may be offered CBT (Cognitive Behavioural Therapy) or medication.

Summary

- The two main drivers of your wake–sleep cycle are adenosine (a chemical that puts you to sleep) and your circadian clock.
- Your primary circadian clock, the one in your head, follows a roughly 24-hour day. In some people it runs fast (larks), in others it runs slow (owls).
- The clock is reset every day by bright morning light.
- When children become teenagers they switch from being larks to becoming owls, which explains why so many prefer to stay up late and get up late. There are evolutionary reasons for this.
- Owls can become more larky by following a number of simple rules.
- One of the main reasons we sleep badly is because of snoring and sleep apnoea. This is caused by too much fat around the neck and the best cure is rapid weight loss.

Shift work and jet lag

So far, we have focused on people who follow the normal pattern of waking and sleeping – people who go to bed at night and get up in the morning. But there is a large and growing section of the population who don't do this. They work at night and sleep, if they can, during the day. If you work in one of the caring professions, as a doctor, nurse, paramedic or care worker, you are expected to work antisocial hours. Taking a job working in transport, communications or construction is also likely to be a sleep killer. What these jobs have in common is that they involve a lot of shift work, being awake when your body is desperate to be asleep.

During my medical training, I was frequently sleep deprived, but I never had to put in the sort of hours that my wife Clare did when she was a junior doctor. She was on a rotation where once a month, after a normal 60-hour working week, she would embark on a weekend shift on the Friday night. She would then work through the weekend until the Tuesday evening, before returning the next day to finish a normal week.

Like other doctors I've talked to, she sometimes got so tired that she experienced visual hallucinations. 'I remember, at the end of one of these marathon weekends, walking down this long, old-fashioned

Victorian corridor in the middle of the night and noticing that the whole corridor was snaking and twisting. I was finding it hard to walk straight and to anyone passing it must've looked as if I was drunk.'

Falling asleep on the job is an occupational hazard if you are a junior doctor. As I mentioned in the introduction, Clare briefly fell asleep while assisting during an operation, although no one seemed to notice (they were probably as tired as she was).

A medical friend of ours, Philip, remembers doing a long weekend, after a busy week, and being called down in the middle of the night to see a patient in Emergency. He sat down on the bed to chat with the patient and the next thing he was aware of was the sound of his bleep going off. He had fallen asleep on the bed, in mid-conversation. The patient had left him a note, saying: 'I've gone home, I'm feeling better and I thought you needed the bed more than I do.'

It is hard to prove that sleep-deprived doctors and nurses are harming patients, though I don't think many of us would want to be operated on by a surgeon who had had less than four hours' sleep the night before. Unlike with pilots, there are no measures in place to ensure that medical staff have had enough sleep. Rather, there is tremendous pressure on junior staff to work far longer than they are paid to do, and well beyond what is legal. I have heard countless stories of junior doctors who are still working impossibly long hours simply because that is seen as the main way to get on.

We are not designed for shift work. Our remote ancestors rose at dawn, went hunting or grubbing for food, spent the hours of daylight largely outside, then retired to their caves for sex and sleep.

Their lives and their all-important internal clocks were almost entirely driven by the movements of the sun.

Then, in the 20th century, we saw the invention of the electric light bulb and the jet engine, both of which had a major impact on our circadian clocks.

The jet engine meant that we were now able to get to the other side of the world in 24 hours, which is way too fast for our ancient body clocks to adjust to; while the creation of intense artificial light meant that not only were teenagers able to stay up until the small hours, but an increasing number (roughly 20%) of the population became shift workers, toiling away when their body clocks were screaming at them to sleep.

Jet lag and shift work have a lot in common. In both cases your internal body clock is thrown out of sync with the external world, and this has a number of unfortunate consequences.

In the case of jet lag, the impact can be unpleasant, but it tends not to be long term (unless you do an awful lot of travelling). For shift workers it can be truly life changing. Fortunately, there are things you can do to make shift work more tolerable, and I will come to those in a moment. First, I want to look at jet lag.

How to overcome jet lag

Lots of flying is bad for the planet and it is not good for the brain. A study found that putting female hamsters on a brief jet lag regime damaged the hippocampus, an area of the brain that is important for learning and memory.[17] The effects on memory persisted for weeks after the jet-lagged hamsters had returned to their normal sleeping pattern.

Jet lag can make you do stupid things. Former US President George W. Bush memorably tried to blame jet lag for an embarrassing press conference in Beijing, which he tried to cut short by attempting to exit through what was plainly a locked door. After tugging repeatedly at the door, he admitted to the gathered press: 'I was trying to escape. Obviously, it didn't work.'

I haven't done anything quite that publicly embarrassing, though I did once manage to walk out of my hotel room in the night, semi-naked, thinking I was heading for the bathroom. By the time I realised what I had done, the door had slammed shut behind me. I had to sneak down to reception and get another key.

Since jet lag is caused by the imbalance between your internal body clock and your new time zone, the journeys that produce the most brutal effect are, not surprisingly, the ones that involve flying through multiple time zones. In my case, that means flights to places like Australia and the US, which I have to do occasionally for business.

Before I found ways of coping, jet lag would leave me feeling dazed, hungry and irritable, madly craving carbs at crazy times of the day and night.

The good news is that there are things you can do to reduce the impact of jet lag. But they require a bit of forward planning.

SLEEPING PILLS AND MELATONIN

If you don't already have them, see if you can get prescriptions for sleeping pills and melatonin from your GP. Although doctors are understandably reluctant to prescribe sleeping pills for long-term use, they are more sympathetic if you just need some to get you through jet lag. I use zopiclone (also known by the brand name Imovane).

As I mentioned on page 49, melatonin is an important hormone for resetting your internal clock. A Cochrane review,[18] which looked at nine studies involving nearly 1000 people, concluded that: 'Melatonin is remarkably effective in preventing or reducing jet lag, and occasional short-term use appears to be safe. It should be recommended to adult travellers flying across five or more time zones, particularly in an easterly direction, and especially if they have experienced jet lag on previous journeys. Travellers crossing 2–4 time zones can also use it if need be.'

I find this pretty convincing as Cochrane reviews are widely regarded as the best when it comes to assessing medical evidence.

THE ARGONNE DIET

Widely used by the US military, this is a way of combatting jet lag created in the 1980s by Dr Charles Ehret, a researcher at the Argonne National Laboratory, near Chicago. Dr Ehret, an expert in circadian rhythms, discovered that you could reset your internal clock faster if, for three days before flying, you alternated feasting and fasting. His regime was simple:

- On day one, a fast day, you have to restrict yourself to 800 calories. You can find suitable recipes in my book, *The Fast 800*, or go to thefast800.com.

- On day two, a feast day, you eat a high-protein breakfast, an above-average-size lunch and have an early dinner. Don't drink coffee after 5pm.

- On day three, the day before your flight, you have another 800-calorie day.

- On the day of your flight, you don't break your fast till your destination breakfast time. In other words, if you are in London, travelling to New York, your first meal of the day would be at 1pm UK time (8am in New York). If you are travelling to Sydney, on the other hand, you would not eat until 7pm.

So does it work? In 2002, the US military decided to put the Argonne diet to the test.[19] They split 186 soldiers, travelling to South Korea for military duties, into two groups; half did the Argonne diet, the others ate normally. It was found that those who had followed the Argonne diet were seven and a half times less likely to experience serious jet lag than those who had eaten normally.

THE FAST VERSION OF THE ARGONNE DIET

If the Argonne diet sounds a bit tough, there is a simplified version you can try, developed by researchers at the Beth Israel Deaconess Medical Center in Boston. It is the one I most commonly use.

The idea is simple: you do a short fast on the day that you fly. It is based on the fact that, like light and darkness, when you eat has a powerful effect on resynchronising your body clocks.

When you are 'fasting' you should drink plenty of water and herbal tea, but no alcohol or caffeine. Below is an example of what I do to minimise jet lag, based on extensive personal experience and lots of chats with air crews and sleep experts.

1. On the day of the flight

Firstly, I always pack a sleeping mask, wax ear plugs, an empty water bottle, noise-cancelling headphones, an inflatable travel pillow and a good book.

If I am heading to New York – five hours behind the UK – I like to get an early-afternoon flight. When I get up, I skip breakfast and aim not to eat anything until at least 1pm (8am New York time).

At the airport, I set my watch to New York time, then walk around a lot.

I do squats and press-ups and use airport chairs to do triceps dips. I also drink a lot of water. I don't drink any alcohol or caffeine in the airport or on the plane.

If I get a 1pm flight, I will normally have a light lunch on the plane, and then nothing more until I have a high-protein evening meal when I get to my hotel in New York (which is normally around 5pm). I go to bed at 9pm, having swallowed a melatonin capsule and a sleeping pill.

2. The next morning

I get up at around 6am and when it is light I go for a 30-minute walk (or run, if I'm feeling particularly energetic). This is partly to get some exercise but also to grab some morning light. Then I have a protein-rich breakfast (omelettes, scrambled eggs, that sort of thing) and get on with my day.

I normally take melatonin on the second night, and sometimes a sleeping pill. I find that within a day or two I can sleep happily without them.

3. Returning home

On the way back to London from the US, I get an early-evening flight, after a good lunch at 2pm. I skip dinner on the plane and, with the aid of melatonin and a sleeping pill, try to get to sleep as quickly as possible. I also skip breakfast on the plane.

When I get back home, after a 14-hour fast, I have breakfast. I go for a brisk mid-morning walk or run, to perk myself up. I have a light lunch, a protein-rich evening meal and go to bed at my normal time, after taking a melatonin capsule and a sleeping pill. This usually works brilliantly.

Q&A

Why is it harder flying east than west?

It is mainly because it is easier to stay up and go to sleep later than normal, rather than go to sleep much earlier than normal. If you have flown west, from London to New York, and it is 9pm in New York, you should find it easy to go to sleep because your internal clock is telling you that it is 2am.

Going east, from New York to the UK, means that when it is 11pm in London your body is telling you it is really only 6pm, so why on earth are you going to bed? That's when I really need a sleeping pill.

What about naps?

Personally, I don't do naps, because I need the build-up of sleep pressure to put me to sleep and keep me asleep. If you find them refreshing then that is fine, but no more than 40 minutes.

How to manage shift work

While jet lag is unpleasant, shift work can be deadly. There is a long list of terrible things that prolonged shift work can do to the human body, ranging from increased risk of heart disease, type 2 diabetes, cancer and obesity, through early menopause to depression and divorce.

One shocking statistic that I came across is that in the US, more firefighters are killed in traffic accidents and from heart attacks than in fires. Although firefighters (like most shift workers) are likely to have a major sleep disorder, few seem to realise it.

A study of 7000 American firefighters[20] found that 37% had at least one major disorder, the most common being obstructive sleep apnoea. The vast majority of them (80%) were undiagnosed and didn't realise that this put them at twice the risk of heart disease or diabetes. They were also more than three times as likely to suffer from depression and anxiety.

A similar study, which looked at American police officers, showed similar results, with around 40% having significant sleep problems.[21]

What is their life like? In the course of researching this book, I had a fascinating chat with Joe, who is 48 years old and has been a firefighter for 18 years. Like most firefighters in the UK, he works two day shifts, followed by two night shifts, then has four days off. On his day shifts, he works from 9am until 6pm, then he does two night shifts, when he works from 6pm until 9am. When he's doing the night shifts, he gets the chance to have a bit of shut-eye, but this is unpredictable, and it is always noisy at the fire station.

Joe is a bit of a foodie, so when he is doing a night shift he tries to eat healthily. He brings his own meals to work, featuring high-protein foods such as poached eggs and smoked salmon. There is a canteen in his fire station, which does provide food, but it is mainly pasta and other high-carb, rather stodgy foods. Unlike most of the others, who often snack, Joe tries not to eat again until lunchtime the next day. He is a fan of time-restricted eating (TRE) and finds that eating during his night shift makes him feel sluggish. If things are quiet, the team are allowed to sleep in a dormitory, but they are expected to be up and out of the building within 90 seconds of the alarm going off. So Joe sleeps lightly, half awake, anticipating the ringing of the alarm: 'I always wake to the soft click, which happens just before the alarm itself goes off.'

After he has returned home from a night shift, Joe prefers not to go to sleep, because this leaves him feeling tired and grumpy. His main way of coping is by doing lots of exercise. He finds doing night shifts has got harder as the years have gone by.

What I found startling, when I talked to firefighters like Joe, to police officers, nurses and paramedics, is that none of them get any specific advice on how to cope with being a shift worker. They are just left to get on with it.

My son Jack is also a shift worker. He is a junior doctor and every few weeks he has to do a couple of nights on call, from 9pm to 9am. Jack has a nap in the afternoon before work, and a meal in the early evening. He also takes food into the hospital to eat before midnight, as the only alternative is something out of a vending machine. And, like Joe, he practises TRE, trying not to eat between midnight and 9am, when he finishes work. Instead, he drinks lots of water and tea.

He also takes a sleeping bag into the hospital with him and, depending on how busy he is, sometimes manages to get a bit of sleep on the floor of the doctors' office. He finds that a short nap in the early hours means he feels less tired when driving home after a night on call.

WHAT CAN YOU DO TO COUNTER THE EFFECTS OF SHIFT WORK?

In recent years, there has been a lot of research into shift work and some things are very clear.[22]

IF YOU ARE AN EMPLOYER:

1. You should be aware that employees over the age of 45 years are less able to adapt to shift work, and the impact on their bodies and brains is greater. I had a chat with Dave, a night-time security guard, who says he relies on Red Bull, junk food and cigarettes to stay awake. He is in his mid-fifties and has put on 15kg since he started doing night work two years ago. He has type 2 diabetes, high blood pressure, sleep apnoea, and gets around five hours' sleep a night. Not surprisingly he often falls asleep at work.

2. If you are creating a shift-work schedule, then do take your employees' chronotype into account. Don't make larks do the late shift, or owls the early shift, if you can avoid it.

3. If your employees have to do a rotational shift, it should always go in a clockwise direction (start them off doing days, then evenings, then nights), because it is much easier to adjust to this than random shifts or shifts that go counter-clockwise.

Do try and provide a place where employees can have a short nap, even if it is only 20 minutes. A study of engineers in New Zealand[23] showed that getting a 20-minute nap during the night shift significantly improved their performance, while a study of American nurses found that a 20-minute nap meant they were less drowsy on their drive home. This study also found that many hospital managers, who don't work nights, are very resistant to providing napping opportunities.

IF YOU ARE A NIGHT SHIFT WORKER:

1. Before your shift begins, take a long nap. If you can, try to get the majority of your sleep in the hours leading up to starting work. There is evidence that if you are working a night shift, say from 11pm to 7am, it is better to have an evening sleep (from 2pm to 9pm) rather than a morning sleep (8am to 3pm). In one study,[24] shift workers who slept in the afternoon made fewer mistakes at work than the morning sleepers.

   If you are driving to work, you should try to wake up at least an hour before heading off as it can take that long to become fully alert.

   Put together a bag with healthy food and drink to take with you. The kind of food available from vending machines is likely to be high in sugar, saturated fat and salt, and low in fibre and nutrients. When you eat junk food you pack in the calories and are soon hungry again. Plus, the fact that you are eating at night, when your body will find it hard to process, means the bad stuff will hang around in your system for longer. So try to eat your main meal before midnight, and take in nuts, apples and pears to snack on if you can't endure a long night without anything.

   Take in a bottle of water, from the fridge, to sip during overnight shifts. Do not drink caffeinated fizzy drinks.

2. While you're at work, during the early hours of your night shift, make sure you are getting some bright light. If the place where you are working is dimly lit, bring in a light box to give yourself a 20-minute blast. It is more effective and certainly healthier than caffeine at night.

Do try TRE. There is a lot of evidence that eating when your body thinks it should be asleep is really bad for the heart. There are a couple of major studies going on at the moment in the US and Australia looking at the benefits of limiting the hours within which you eat while doing an overnight shift. Researchers from Monash University, for example, are asking people to avoid eating between 1am and 6am, to see what impact that has on their risk of heart disease.[25]

If you get the chance, and there is somewhere you can safely do it, get in a 20- to 40-minute nap at some point during your shift.

3. When you are travelling home after a night shift, try to car-share, take public transport, walk or cycle. If you have to drive, a short nap before heading off in the car may also help.

On the journey home, you could try wearing dark glasses. The idea is to avoid morning light, where possible.

Some people go straight to bed when they get home, and if you have a family with young children, this makes sense because they will probably be at school. However, research so far shows that sleeping in the afternoon seems to be better.

To get a decent sleep, you will probably need wax ear plugs or white noise, a sleep mask and a prominent 'Do Not Disturb' sign on the bedroom door. You will also need to follow the sleep hygiene tips I recommended in Chapter 5: i.e. have a fixed time when you go to sleep and wake up; a strict countdown to your bedtime routine; no caffeine or alcohol before bedtime, etc.

WILL TAKING MELATONIN HELP?

The short answer is that it may. The Cochrane reviewers concluded that the use of melatonin by night shift workers increased the amount of sleep they got by 24 minutes.

DO ALL SHIFT WORKERS HAVE PROBLEMS?

No. There are some people who cope well with shift work, but being older and female seems to make it harder to adapt. Apart from the impact on your body, it can also mess with your personal life. If you or your partner are shift workers, you are six times more likely to get divorced than if you work days.[26]

One of the reasons for such high rates of divorce is that shift workers find it hard to take part in 'normal' family life and plan family events.

As Sue, a nurse who works nights, told me: 'Working nights means you have time at home, in the day, so it's great for going to the bank or shopping. The trouble is that most school events, like plays or meeting teachers, happen in the evening. My husband, who is a paramedic, also works nights. We leave each other notes in the kitchen, but sometimes it feels like days go by without us really talking to each other.'

People who don't adapt soon develop a condition called Shift Work Sleep Disorder (SWSD). Common symptoms of SWSD include:

- Feeling excessively sleepy, both on and off the job;
- Having difficulty concentrating;
- Finding it hard to go to sleep and waking up feeling tired;
- Feeling depressed or moody;

- Having trouble with close relationships, such as with friends and family.

If you are a shift worker, and you think you might have SWSD, and none of the things I've suggested help, do go and see your doctor. You may be prescribed sleeping pills, melatonin or modafinil.

Modafinil is a wake-promoting drug, widely used by the American military to keep their troops alert. Its main medical use is to treat narcolepsy, a rare brain condition that causes people to suddenly fall asleep at inappropriate times. People with narcolepsy I've interviewed have told me extraordinary stories of falling asleep on rollercoasters, in the middle of dinner or even when out riding a horse.

Studies have shown that taking 200mg of modafinil an hour before a night shift can significantly improve your performance without affecting your sleep the following day.[27] As well as perking you up, modafinil has been shown to reduce long-term memory damage in shift workers with SWSD.

Modafinil is a prescription-only drug, but it has far more side effects than melatonin. Despite this, it is widely, and illegally, used as a cognitive enhancer or 'smart drug'. It is particularly popular with university students; surveys suggest that up to 20% use it around exam time. However, taking modafinil in the hope that it will improve your exam results is almost certainly counterproductive; a recent study conducted with healthy volunteers showed that students taking modafinil did worse in memory and cognitive tests than students taking placebo pills.[28]

I took modafinil a few years ago as part of a sleep deprivation experiment and it certainly kept me wide awake. However, as I've just pointed out, modafinil can have significant side effects, including the risk of developing an allergic reaction. Which is what happened to me. I developed such a severe allergic reaction that I had to go to hospital, where they gave me a big dose of steroids to dampen down my immune system. In retrospect, it is one of the scariest self-experiments I have done. So, never again.

Summary

- Problems with jet lag and shift work are caused by the fact that your circadian clock is out of sync with the world outside. You are trying to sleep when your body clock is saying you should be awake, and vice versa.
- Jet lag can be improved by following either the Argonne diet or a modified version which requires a 14-hour fast.
- The rule is that you don't eat until the equivalent of breakfast time at your destination. So if you are flying from London to New York, you skip breakfast and don't eat until at least 1pm (8am New York time).
- Doing this will help speed up how quickly your body is able to adjust to local time.
- Shift work is harder to treat, but there are things that can help, such as having your main sleep in the hours running up to work and trying to practise TRE while at work.

4. Are you getting enough?

Sleep is essential for spring-cleaning our brains, putting our memories into long-term storage and boosting creativity. Poor sleep, as we saw in Chapter 1, contributes to low mood, obesity, type 2 diabetes and low sex drive.[29]

Far from being 'a criminal waste of time', as the inventor Thomas Edison claimed, getting enough good-quality sleep is vital for our mental and physical well-being. But how do you know if you are getting enough?

According to the National Sleep Foundation, these are the targets you should be hitting at different stages of your life:

Age	Recommended hours' sleep
1–12 mths	14–15 hours
1–3 years	12–14 hours
3–6 years	10–12 hours
7–12 years	10–11 hours
12–18 years	8–9 hours
18–65 years	7–9 hours
65+ years	7–8 hours

Most modern teenagers don't come close to hitting these targets, with fewer than half of British or American kids getting the required hours. Computer-crazed South Korean teenagers do even worse, with the average 17-year-old student managing just 5.7 hours a night.[30]

Adults get closer to their targets than teenagers, though according to a recent Gallup survey,[31] the average adult in the US still gets only 6.8 hours a night. That is a full hour less than adults said they were getting in 1942.

Surveys conducted in the UK come up with similar figures.

A couple of years ago I helped set up The UK SLEEP CENSUS, with the University of Oxford's Sleep and Circadian Neuroscience Institute. More than 200,000 people answered our online survey, and the ones who completed the census reported sleeping for just 6 hours 48 minutes, on average.

Forty-four per cent of them also reported having poor quality sleep, and this was linked with low mood, cognitive problems, and a poorer quality of life. Those who said they had problems sleeping also said the thoughts that kept them awake included worrying about their responsibilities, thinking about the future and reflecting on things that had happened that day.

When it comes to sleep Australians do slightly better, hitting an average of seven hours and 18 minutes.[32]

Bear in mind that 'sleep' in this context really means 'hours in bed'. Since even good sleepers spend around 15% of their time in bed awake, if you are in bed for seven hours you are probably getting less than six hours' actual sleep a night. The other thing about taking an 'average' figure is that some people need more than average, while others will need less.

So how do you know if you are getting enough sleep? You could fill in a questionnaire, such as the Pittsburgh Sleep Quality Index, which you can find online, but I prefer the simplicity of the Sleep Onset Latency Test.

The Sleep Onset Latency Test or Spoon Test

The idea behind this test is to see how quickly you fall asleep during the day, if you are given a chance. Daytime sleepiness is a good measure of 'sleep debt' and therefore of whether you are getting enough good-quality sleep at night. If you fall asleep while watching TV or at the cinema then you probably have 'sleep debt'.

The great thing about this test is that it doesn't require any fancy lab equipment; you just need a metal spoon and a metal tray. The version

I'm about to describe was developed by a famous sleep researcher, Professor Nathaniel Kleitman, from the University of Chicago.

At the weekend, or whenever is most convenient, you skip your usual morning coffee or tea. Then, in the early afternoon, any time between 1pm and 3pm, you go to your bedroom with a metal spoon and a metal tray.

You close the curtains, place the metal tray on the floor by your bed, check the time, then hang your arm over the side of the bed, clutching the spoon. Finally, you close your eyes and try to drift off.

The idea is that if you fall asleep, the spoon will drop from your fingers and hit the tray with a loud clang, waking you up. As soon as that happens, you check your watch to see how much time has passed.

- If you fall asleep within five minutes of closing your eyes, it means you are severely sleep deprived.
- Falling asleep within five to ten minutes is deemed to be 'troublesome'.
- Falling asleep after 10–15 minutes suggests you have a mild problem.
- If you stay awake for over 15 minutes, you're probably fine.

An alternative version of this test, which is more practical but less fun, is to go to bed in the afternoon, as described, but this time you just set an alarm on your phone to go off after 15 minutes. You then see if you drop off before the alarm goes off.

I told a friend, Sarah, about the spoon test and she decided to give it a go. Sarah normally goes to bed around midnight and wakes up at 5am. She lies quietly for an hour or so, just listening to the sounds around her, and then gets up quite happily.

Because she had read so much about the importance of getting at least seven hours' sleep a night, she wondered if she was doing something wrong. Anyway, she did the spoon test and passed it with flying colours. As I said to her afterwards, she must be one of those relatively rare people who can get by on less than five hours' sleep without having any obvious problems.

Her husband also did the test. He fell asleep within 10 minutes.

The Multiple Sleep Latency Test

This is a more sophisticated version of the above, normally carried out in a sleep lab.

When you arrive at the lab, you are attached to numerous machines (to record brainwaves, eye movements, muscle tone, etc.) and asked to lie down in a dark, quiet room during the day. The scientists measure how quickly you fall asleep and how deeply. After 20 minutes you are woken up. Then, two hours later, you do it again. And then again. In fact, you do this a total of five times. This test is used to diagnose whether you have a sleep problem, and if so what type. Do you have narcolepsy or idiopathic hypersomnolence? A breathing disorder or excessive daytime sleepiness? It is expensive, but it is the most reliable way of getting to the root of a persistent sleep problem.

Who is the most sleep deprived?

TEENAGERS

Most teenagers need between eight and ten hours in bed each night, but as we have seen, in many countries, including the US and the UK, less than half are getting the amount of sleep required by their growing bodies and brains. That is why I am a great believer in moving the school day later, to fit in with their owl-like tendencies. Lack of sleep limits teenagers' ability to concentrate and learn new facts, and it also leads to aggressive and risky behaviour. One study[33] found that teens who average less than seven hours a night were twice as likely to have unsafe sex than those sleeping for longer.

Sleep-deprived teenagers also eat more junk food. This makes them overweight, anxious and depressed, which makes their sleep even worse. Being sympathetic and helping your teenager improve their sleep hygiene (see Chapter 5) will make a big difference to family life.

PARENTS WITH YOUNG CHILDREN

As anyone who has had kids will know, you spend the first few months after they are born wandering around like a zombie in the middle of the night, warming up milk and trying to stop them crying. If that sounds bad, then listen to this: according to a recent study by Warwick University,[34] it takes new parents at least six years to get back to sleeping as well as they did before having children.

For this particular study, the researchers asked 4659 would-be parents to keep a record of how well they slept prior to the birth of their child, and then followed them for six years.

Mums lost an average of one hour's sleep a night for the first three months after giving birth, while dads struggled by with a loss of just 15 minutes' sleep a night. Although things got slowly better, by the time their child was six years old, mums were still sleeping 20 minutes less than they had before pregnancy, while fathers were still having to make do with 15 minutes less. Both sexes were significantly less happy with the quality of their sleep than they had been before becoming parents.

First-time parents were the most affected, probably because they tend to be more conscientious. When our oldest son was born, we both leapt out of bed every time he whimpered. By the time our youngest child came on the scene, we were more inclined to let her settle herself, and she did.

The best thing to be said about this phase of life is 'it will pass'.

OLDER PEOPLE

Sleep deprivation becomes a bigger problem as we get older, with more than half of those over the age of 65 saying they have difficulty getting a good night's sleep. It is a myth that older people need less sleep. They need just as much, but most don't get it. Although you have more time on your hands when you retire, and one would imagine fewer responsibilities, as people get older they snore more and need to get up in the night more often to go to the loo. Older people also take more medication, which can interfere with sleep, and the quality of their microbiome (gut bacteria) tends to deteriorate. As we'll see, the microbiome can have a big impact on sleep (see Chapter 6).

MENOPAUSAL WOMEN

The menopause and its aftermath can trigger severe insomnia. Around 60% of post-menopausal women report occasional insomnia. Snoring and OSA are also much more common after the menopause.[35]

So, why does it happen and what, if anything, can you do about it?

The frustrating thing for many women, particularly those in their 40s, is they start gaining extra pounds without any obvious change in lifestyle. One, of course, of the main factors is the sudden change in hormones that occurs around the menopause.

As oestrogen levels drop, women are more likely to gain weight around their stomachs, rather than their hips or thighs (exactly why is unknown).

Hormonal changes also mean that sleep gets worse, which drives hunger and cravings – in particular, for energy-dense (i.e.calorific) foods.

A little known, but highly effective way to counter a tendency to overeat is to boost your protein intake – because protein is more satiating than fat or carbs and your body uses more energy to break it down. Work by two leading Australian researchers, Professor David Raubenheimer and Professor Steve Simpson, experts in the dietary causes of obesity – suggest that many menopausal women could benefit from eating more protein. They say one of the reasons for middle-age weight gain is because when women enter the menopause, their need for protein rises, and unless they do something about this they are likely to get hungrier than normal and compensate by eating more junk food.

But there is good news. In a recent paper, published in a journal of the Royal College of Obstetricians and Gynaecologists, the two scientists say that to stop this, all you need to do is boost your protein intake by a few per cent. If you put aside that sugary snack and instead eat more protein-rich foods, such as eggs, meat, fish, beans or tofu, you will experience less hunger and fewer cravings.

Boosting protein intake in middle age should not only help stop substantial weight gain, but also reduce the risk of osteoporosis and sarcopenia (loss of muscle mass), as protein is vital for maintaining strong bones and muscles.

This doesn't only apply to women going through the menopause – it also affects men beyond the age of 60. So why do our protein needs change? With the menopause it seems that the fall in oestrogen leads to increased breakdown of protein stored as tissue in your body.

But it is also because as we get older our bodies (male or female) become less efficient at absorbing and using protein.

Protein is also a big driver of hunger. The professors demonstrated this in an elegant experiment a few years ago, where they recruited 22 healthy volunteers and kept them locked away in hotel-style accommodation at Sydney University.

The volunteers were given meals and snacks matched for calories, but containing different amounts of protein. It made a big difference.

Without realising it participants ate, on average, 210 calories more per day when on the lower-protein diet than the higher-protein one.

They also felt far hungrier a couple of hours after eating the low-protein breakfast. That is certainly what I find. When I eat eggs or kippers for breakfast, I stay full until lunchtime. If I eat the same number of calories in the form of cereal or toast, I am craving a snack by mid-morning.

In part, that is because eating protein reduces levels of the hunger hormone ghrelin, while boosting levels of a hormone called peptide YY, which makes you feel full.

Standard guidelines say women should be aiming to eat about 45g of protein a day, and men, 55g. But many experts think these numbers are too low, particularly when we get older. According to the International Osteoporosis Foundation, eating more protein 'is associated with higher bone density, a slower rate of bone loss and reduced risk of hip fracture.'[36]

And a large US study called the Framingham Heart Study Offspring found that, over a two-decade period, those who ate at least 90g of protein a day scored better on measures of frailty, including grip strength, being able to go up and down stairs, walk half a mile or dress themselves, than those who had 60g or less a day.

HOW TO BOOST PROTEIN

Research suggests that your body absorbs more protein if you spread your intake across the day, rather than having it in just one meal – and that a protein-rich breakfast is a particularly good way to prevent hunger later in the day.

So why not start your day with eggs? I often have two for breakfast (14g of protein), with smoked salmon (a 60g portion provides 11g protein), or sometimes bacon (a rasher has around 8g protein). See our recipes on pages 224–92.

And if you're worried about eggs and your heart, a 2018 study in the journal *Heart*, which included half a million adults, found people who ate eggs most days had a lower risk of heart disease and stroke than those who ate eggs less frequently. Porridge, made with rolled oats (rather than the instant stuff), is a good source of protein, particularly when made with cow's milk and with nuts sprinkled on top, providing 14g in half a cup.

Eating Greek yoghurt is also a good way to top up your protein levels, particularly if you sprinkle over a few nuts. I think this yoghurt tastes better and because it's strained, typically contains about twice the amount of protein, about 12g in half a cup.

For lunch, or your evening meal, a serving of beef, pork or chicken will give you a protein boost, delivering 33g of protein for every 100g of meat. Or you might prefer fish, with a small piece of salmon adding up to roughly 30g of protein.

Along with fish or meat, why not give quinoa a go? It is a trendy food, which many people think is a grain, like rice, but it's actually a seed. Although quinoa is more expensive than rice, my wife Clare and I eat it fairly often because it's rich in fibre and minerals, but also because it contains around 8g of protein per 50g serving. If you're a vegetarian, or simply want a break from meat, then beans and lentils are protein packed.

One cup of cooked lentils (200g) provides around 20g of protein, while tofu, which is a great meat substitute, gives you about 18g of protein per 150g.

Following the recipes and advice that I outline in the 4-Week Sleep Plan is a very effective way of treating insomnia in post-menopausal women, but taking Hormone Replacement Therapy (HRT) can also help. A randomised controlled trial[37] in which more than 400 post-menopausal women aged between 50 and 69 were given HRT or a placebo found that those taking HRT reported significantly less insomnia as well as fewer hot flushes, night sweats, aching joints and vaginal dryness. You can get HRT in the form of pills, patches, gels or creams.

Why do we need to sleep as much as we do?

We know that not getting enough sleep has a big impact on your brain and your body. But why most of us need at least 6–7 hours of sleep each night is more of a mystery.

Horses, giraffes and elephants seem to get by quite happily on a couple of hours, while our fellow primates need considerably more than we do. Orangutans curl up in a bed in the fork of a tree, and get a solid 10 hours, snoring away sweetly like a great, hairy, orange baby. Baboons, on the other hand, sleep on their bottoms while balancing on a branch high above the forest floor. They also sleep for around 10 hours a night, though their sleep is rather more fragmented.

Some anthropologists think that the invention of the bed (or, more accurately, 'a sleeping platform') by great apes, tens of millions of years ago, was a hugely important part of our evolutionary story.

Sleeping platforms meant that, unlike the precarious baboons, our remote ancestors could sleep securely in the trees, safe from predators and blood-sucking insects. It also allowed them to get more deep and REM sleep, which presumably boosted their brain power.

But if sleep is so important for brain development, why do humans, with the biggest brains of all the primates, sleep the least? The short answer is: nobody knows. One thing's for certain: the amount of sleep you need is not related to the size of your intellect. In our house we have a dog and a cat, and they spend at least half their lives sleeping. No one who's met either would describe them as particularly smart.

How long can you go without any sleep?

In 1983, Allan Rechtschaffen and colleagues from the University of Chicago reported the results of a gruesome sleep deprivation experiment they had performed on rats.[38]

They took eight rats and put them in a cage with a pool of water at the bottom. The rats could keep dry by standing on a metal disk. But as soon as they showed signs of falling asleep, the disk would rotate, so they had to scamper to stop falling into the water. Within a few days, the sleep-deprived rats had swollen paws, and were losing their balance and starting to lose weight. Within a few weeks, they were all dead. Yet when they were dissected no obvious cause of death was found.

Sleep deprivation has been widely used as a form of torture but, as far as I know, no equivalent of the rat study has ever been done on humans. Thanks to an unfortunate Italian family, however, we have a good idea about what happens when humans are deprived of sleep for a long time. It isn't pretty.

The story begins in the early 1970s when an Italian physician, Dr Ignazio Roiter, living in a small town in northern Italy, was asked by his wife, Elisabetta, to examine her aunt. The unfortunate aunt had stopped sleeping and started to experience terrible hallucinations. They tried all sorts of drugs to put her to sleep but nothing worked. Over the next few months she remained sleepless; her body wasted away, until eventually she died. No one could explain what had happened, so the family, though upset and puzzled, mourned and moved on.

Then another of Elisabetta's aunts began to show the same strange symptoms. She found it harder and harder to sleep until she stopped sleeping altogether. She eventually died the same horrible death.

Dr Roiter began to investigate his wife's family tree and discovered that the same thing had happened to generations of Elisabetta's family, going back into the early 19th century.

When Elisabetta's Uncle Silvano started to develop signs of severe insomnia, Dr Roiter put him in contact with a sleep specialist, who was unable to do anything to help him.

After Uncle Silvano died, his brain was sent to experts in the US, who finally discovered that Silvano, like so many other members of the family, had died from a disorder which was later called Fatal Familial Insomnia (FFI). It is a genetic disease where the body starts to produce an abnormal protein, called a prion protein, which slowly attacks and destroys the thalamus, an area of the brain which is partly responsible for regulating sleep. The good news is that a genetic test is now available. The bad news is that there is no cure and, if you have the abnormal gene, there is nothing anyone can do to prevent you falling into a twilight world of perpetual insomnia which ultimately leads to insanity and death.

Going for broke

Unlike Dr Rechtschaffen's rats and families with FFI, there are some people crazy enough to voluntarily go without sleep for long, long periods of time.

The official record for staying awake was set in 1964 by a 17-year-old high-school student called Randy Gardner. He wanted to win the Greater San Diego School Science prize and he thought breaking the world record would be one way to do that.

In a recent interview,[39] he said the first two days were OK, but by day three he was moody and uncoordinated. By day five he had started to hallucinate. Tests showed he was having trouble concentrating and forming short-term memories. Despite this he kept going. Finally, after 11 days, he'd had enough. He was driven to a local hospital where he was fitted with an EEG and then allowed to sleep.

He slept for 14 hours, for much of which he was in REM sleep. He was kept in the hospital for a couple more days, then went back to school. His self-experiment won him the coveted science prize.

There were no obvious side effects at the time, but years later, when Randy was in his sixties, he developed severe insomnia, which he describes as 'karmic payback'. He still struggles with his sleep.

Although Randy holds the *official* record of 264 hours, others have gone longer. In 2007, Tony Wright, a Cornish gardener, managed to stay awake for 266 hours, while being filmed in a bar in Penzance. He passed the time by drinking tea, playing pool and keeping a diary. His achievement is not in the Guinness World Records because the publishers don't want to encourage others to try to beat it.

I met Tony a few years ago, when I was making a documentary about sleep. Among other things, I wanted to see how long I could stay awake and what effect it would have on me. I asked Tony to join in, to give me tips and moral support.

Before starting, we did some cognitive tests (test of memory, mood, reaction times, etc.) and then, after a decent night's sleep, we began what I think is the most challenging stunt I have ever attempted (and I've done quite a few).

The first 24 hours weren't too bad, though the tests we were doing showed that I was already falling apart. My reaction times had slowed right down, I had become intensely irritable and I was starving hungry. When I did a car-driving simulation test, I kept on crashing.

Tony, however, was holding up remarkably well. He did fine on the car-driving simulation test and his reaction times, grip strength and balance showed no signs of deteriorating. His mood was good and, if anything, he became more cheerful as the hours dragged by.

I struggled on, feeling more and more dreadful. I kept myself going by pacing around, singing and playing pool. Neither of us was allowed caffeinated drinks or any form of stimulant.

There were peaks and troughs. We were in New York (the producer liked the idea of filming a programme about not sleeping in the City That Never Sleeps), and I remember vividly, after 48 hours of being awake, the wonderful feeling of standing beside the river in Brooklyn and watching dawn rise over the city of Manhattan. The rising sun touched something inside me. My mood lifted and I felt gloriously alive.

The reason for this little burst of euphoria was that while the pressure to sleep, coming from the build-up of adenosine in my brain, was still increasing steadily, the start of a new day meant that my circadian clock was now insisting that I wake up and get on with my life. For a few hours, these two systems battled away, with my circadian clock slightly on top, but by mid-afternoon I was feeling truly shattered and had to fight to keep my eyes open. We went off to play baseball and my reaction times were now so bad I missed the ball every time. Tony was in excellent form and smashed the ball all over the place.

When the sun set, I had such a feeling of dread that I knew I couldn't go on much longer. My blood pressure was up, my blood sugar had soared, I had a thundering headache and I performed badly on all the tests, particularly anything involving concentration or memory.

Tony remained annoyingly cheerful, and did his best to rally me, but by around 11pm I told him and the producer that I couldn't continue. I had begun to hallucinate that the hotel walls were caving in. I staggered up to my bed and took a final look at my watch. I had managed a miserly 64 hours without sleep.

As soon as my head hit the pillow, I was asleep. I slept for 10 hours, and woke up feeling absolutely fine. So why couldn't I go even three days without collapsing, while Tony had managed more than 11? He said he thought it was a combination of his diet and his training. He had put himself on what he called a 'Stone Age' diet, consisting mainly of raw food, and he was convinced that this helped.

I wondered if he, rather like a dolphin, might have the ability to sleep on different sides of his brain, allowing him to appear partly awake while being partly asleep.

This is not completely crazy. A team from Boston recently found that on their first night in a sleep lab,[40] most people show signs on the EEG of being much more deeply asleep on the right side of the brain than the left. To see if the left side of the brain really was more alert than the right, the researchers made a noise. The EEG showed that the sleepers had detected the noise, but only on the left-hand side of their brain. The right-hand hemisphere continued in blissfully deep sleep.

It certainly makes sense, from an evolutionary perspective, that when you are sleeping in a new environment you might want to have part of your brain alert, in case there are predators around, while allowing the other half to have a good night's rest. But in humans it only seems to happen in the very short term. By the second night in the sleep lab, researchers found that both sides of the sleepers' brains were just as deeply asleep.

Sleep mutants

I think a more likely explanation for people like Tony is that he is one of those exceptional individuals who are highly resistant to the pressures of sleep. They are rare, but they exist.

In August 2019, researchers from the University of California[41] announced that they had found a family with a genetic mutation that let them live quite happily on four hours' sleep a night. This family have a mutation in a gene called ADRB1, which alters activity in various regions of the brain that regulate sleep.

When the researchers bred rats with the same mutation, the rats slept for nearly an hour a day less than normal rats and it didn't seem to do them any harm. But the fact that short-sleep mutations are rare in humans suggests it might have a downside, otherwise you would expect more of us to be able, like Tony, to get by on four hours a night.

A few more things that happen when you don't get enough sleep

I've mentioned the effects of poor sleep on your memory, your mood, your weight and your risk of getting dementia. But what worried me most about the fact that Clare was working insane hours as a junior doctor was the fact that she was driving home from the hospital afterwards.

FALLING ASLEEP AT THE WHEEL

In a recent survey[42] of more than a thousand British doctors, 40% admitted falling asleep at the wheel after a night shift, and more than one in four said they knew of a colleague who had died in a car accident after a night on call.

We have strict laws against drink-driving, but not against sleep-deprived driving. In the US, sleep-deprived drivers are responsible for an estimated 100,000 car accidents every year and over 1500 deaths. The impact that a bad night's sleep has on your chance of having an accident is dramatic. A recent investigation by the US Department of Transportation[43] found that drivers who'd had four hours or less sleep the night before were 15 times more likely to be involved in a car crash than those who'd had at least seven hours. Someone who is seriously sleep deprived is as dangerous as a drink driver who is well over the legal limit.

In this study, just a little bit more sleep made a massive difference. Those who'd managed to get in five hours before hitting the road were 'only' twice as likely to crash, while those with a good six hours under their belt were a mere 30% more likely to cause a pile-up than those who'd managed seven hours.

Many of us will, at some point, find ourselves falling asleep at the wheel. At least half the people I've quizzed admit to having done it. I do a lot of travelling and on more than one occasion I've been driving home, late at night, fighting to stay awake.

So what should you do if it happens to you?

The best thing would be to find a hotel for the night. If you can't find somewhere to stay, the next best thing is strong coffee and a quick nap. I usually stop at the nearest service station, buy a strong black coffee and drink it. I then set my phone to wake me in 20 minutes, lie back in the car and have a quick snooze.

The caffeine usually takes about 20 minutes to hit my brain, so when I'm woken by my alarm I am already buzzing. I don't drive straight off, but instead go for a stroll and make sure I really am awake before getting back in the car.

Studies have shown that a cup of black coffee, followed by a 20-minute snooze, will make you far more alert than either just having the coffee or just having the snooze.

The downside is you will probably arrive at your destination still buzzing with caffeine and find it hard to go to sleep. Better that than not arriving at all.

WHEN THE CLOCKS CHANGE

Twice a year, every year, 1.5 billion people in 70 countries turn their clocks forward by an hour in the spring and back by an hour in the autumn. This translates into roughly 40 minutes more, or less, sleep, on the night of the change. The effects of this natural experiment are impressive.

First, changing the clocks alters your risk of having a heart attack. In a recent study,[44] researchers looked at the number of people admitted to hospitals throughout the state of Michigan with symptoms of a heart attack on the day after the clocks went forward or back. Moving the clocks forward led to a 24% increase in heart attack admissions, while moving them back resulted in a 21% reduction.

Secondly, you're more likely to have a car accident. A study published in the *New England Journal of Medicine* in 1996[45] found an 8% increase in accidents on the Monday following the clock change.

The clock change could also put you in jail. In a study with the wonderful title 'Sleepy Punishers Are Harsh Punishers',[46] researchers combed through the archives and found that judges in the US give defendants longer sentences the day after switching to daylight-saving time compared to other days of the year. And what applies to grumpy judges applies to the rest of us. Deprive us of sleep and we become harsher and more judgemental.

Summary

- The amount of sleep you need varies hugely, depending on your genes and your age.
- Some adults can get by on less than five hours a night, but most of us can't.
- The most reliable way to tell if you are getting enough sleep is to lie down in a quiet room in the afternoon and see how quickly you fall asleep. If you fall asleep within 10 minutes of closing your eyes, it suggests you're seriously sleep deprived.
- In addition to the long-term impact of sleep deprivation on your brain and body, one of the biggest risks you face after even a single bad night's sleep is having a car crash. Your judgement and reaction times deteriorate without you noticing.

5. Tried and tested ways to improve your sleep

Getting a good night's sleep is crucial for mental and physical well-being, but how important is it to you? What are you prepared to do to get up feeling refreshed in the morning? How much are you prepared to change? Many of us are so used to being chronically tired that we've forgotten what it feels like to be fully rested.

The Spoon Test, or Sleep Onset Latency Test, which I described on page 89, is one good way of assessing whether you are getting enough sleep. I've come across lots of people who don't think they have an issue but who, nonetheless, fail this test when challenged.

Here's another good test to try, which doesn't involve making time to go to bed during the day. Answer 'yes' or 'no' to the following eight questions:

1. When your head hits the pillow do you find it hard to go to sleep?
2. Do you wake up during the night and then find it hard to get back to sleep?
3. Do you wake up earlier than you want to and find it hard to get back to sleep?
4. When you wake up, do you feel exhausted?
5. Do you feel tired and irritable during the day?
6. Do you find it difficult to concentrate during the day because you're feeling tired?
7. Do you get mad cravings for carbs (biscuits, cakes or something sweet) during the day?
8. Do you nod off while watching TV, while in the cinema or in a public place?

If you answer 'yes' to three or more of these questions, it is likely that you have a significant sleep problem, i.e. insomnia. And, as I explained in the introduction, once you've developed insomnia, you are caught up in the cogs of a vicious cycle.

Insomnia changes your brain chemistry so that when you go to bed your brain is overactive and stops you sleeping. Or you fall asleep but wake up in the night, usually to go to the loo – after which you struggle to resettle.

When you return to bed, you find it hard to get back to sleep because your sleep drive has reduced and your thoughts are now galloping around like a wild horse, ricocheting from one anxiety-inducing subject to another.

Although you will, eventually, drift off, when you wake in the morning you feel shattered. So you drink lots of coffee. But the trouble with coffee is that you develop a tolerance to it. So you drink more, or move on to something stronger (like an energy drink). This gets you through the day, but by the time you get home from work you feel exhausted. Despite your good intentions, you really don't want to take the dog for a walk or go to the gym. What you want to do is collapse on the sofa with a glass of wine.

After a late dinner, you nod off on the sofa while watching TV. You wake up, have a final glass of wine and a bit of cheese before heading for bed. But as you go up the stairs, you realise that you no longer feel quite so tired. The nap you had on the sofa has depleted your sleep drive. So when you get into bed, you spend the next half-hour scrolling through social media or news click-bait.

Your partner falls asleep and starts snoring. You turn off the lights, but immediately start thinking about all the things you have to do tomorrow, and how important it is to get a good night's sleep. You begin to worry and fret ...

Does this sound familiar? If so, then Sleep Restriction Therapy (SRT) could be for you. I am going to explain how you do SRT in full in Chapter 7, as part of my 4-Week Sleep Plan. But the principles are simple: for a few weeks, you deliberately *reduce* the amount of time you spend in bed to ensure that when you do go to bed at night you are really tired. Which means you should fall asleep quickly, stay in deep sleep for longer and wake up less frequently during the night.

Critically, sleep restriction will break down the associations in your brain between 'bed' and 'bad sleep'. These beliefs, whether they are conscious or unconscious, are playing a large part in stopping you from getting a good night's sleep. Think of it as a way of getting rid of a bad habit that you have fallen into.

Sleep restriction is the most radical and challenging part of the 4-Week Sleep Plan. The other key elements are:

- Eating to establish a 'sleepy biome';
- Improving your sleep hygiene – your sleep environment (i.e. your bedroom) and your habits around sleep.

If you've read my book, *The Clever Guts Diet*, you will know just how fascinated I am by the microbiome, the trillions of microbes that live in our guts. We've known for some time how important these microbes are for controlling our immune system and our appetite. Now there is new and very compelling evidence that they also have a big role to play in regulating stress and how we sleep.

Among the thousand different species that live in their dark lair in the large intestine there are 'good' ones and 'bad' ones. The good ones, also known as the 'Old Friends', have evolved with us over hundreds of thousands of years, and work hard to keep us healthy. Among other things they manufacture 95% of the body's serotonin. Serotonin is known as the 'feel-good hormone', because it contributes to our sense of well-being and happiness.

As well as affecting our mood, serotonin plays a role in regulating appetite, digestion, sleep and sexual desire. Unfortunately, our guts also harbour plenty of 'bad' microbes, microbes that create inflammation, contributing to anxiety, depression, weight gain ... and sleepless nights.

The good news is you can swiftly change the mix of microbes that live in your gut by changing what you eat. In the next chapter, I will show you how.

Before that, though, we are going to look at other tried and tested ways to help you sleep better. I'm going to take you through a typical 24-hour day, showing you lots of things you can do to improve your 'sleep hygiene', including how to establish good bedtime habits, how to define your optimum sleep window, and how to use mindfulness and breathing exercises to ward off the anxiety and negative thoughts which are the enemy of a good night's rest.

A note of caution: if you have mild sleep problems then putting the following recommendations into practice will help. But if you have proper insomnia they won't be enough. To properly reboot your brain and cure insomnia you will probably also need to do a short course of Sleep Restriction Therapy (SRT) (see Chapter 7). The good news is that, once you've done SRT (and it should take no more than a few weeks) and cracked your insomnia, then you will find that eating gut-friendly foods and practising the following sleep tips will stop you falling back into a world of sleeplessness.

Establishing good bedtime habits

The tricky thing about sleep is that it is such an individual thing. The amount, quality and type of sleep needed vary not only from person to person, but also within each person's lifetime. No one size fits all.

That said, all the experts I've spoken to are passionate about the importance of treating sleep as a habit, one that you can improve with practice, and they all agree that getting into a regular wake-up-go-to-bed routine is a good starting point.

Your regular wake-up-go-to-bed routine is known as your 'sleep window'. I normally go to bed at 11pm, getting up at 7am, and I aim to do this seven days a week. That's my sleep window. If you are an owl, you would, undoubtedly, be happier going to bed later and getting up later. But for people who have children, or who have to work normal hours, getting up much later than 7am isn't practical.

If you don't have young kids, and if you can persuade your boss to allow you to start your day a bit later, then do. You could try explaining that you can't help it, that you are a genetic owl and you will not only be happier but more productive if you are allowed a more flexible working week. If that doesn't work, try converting yourself into a lark (see page 54).

For shift workers, setting a sleep window is also going to be tricky (see Chapter 3 for tips on this). For the rest of us it should be doable.

The really hard part of having a sleep window is sticking to it, particularly at weekends. The temptation will be to sleep in, especially if you have had a late night. But if you are serious about wanting to sort out your sleep, then I'm afraid a lie-in is a temptation you are going to have to resist. The idea that you can catch up, over the weekend, on poor sleep during the week is a total myth.

Part of the problem with a long weekend lie-in is that you will interfere with your circadian rhythms, which play such an important role in driving the urge to sleep.

If you normally go to bed at 11pm during the week but decide to stay up till 2am on a Saturday night, and then get up three hours later on the Sunday morning, that will really throw your circadian clock out of sync. This is the social jet lag I talked about in Chapter 2.

The other problem is that if you get up on Sunday at 10am, and then head to bed and try to sleep at 11pm, you may struggle because you will have a reduced sleep drive. You've been awake for three hours less than during the week, so there will be much less of an adenosine build-up in your brain urging you to go to sleep.

Obviously, there are nights when you will want to go out on the town but the critical thing is that once you decide the time that you are going to get up in the morning, you stick to it.

CLEARING OUT THE BEDROOM JUNK

One of my top tips for anyone who is about to go on a diet is, before they start, to clear their cupboards of tempting treats and unhealthy foods. If there are crisps, biscuits or chocolate in our house, despite everything I know about how bad these foods are for my brain and my waistline, I will eat them. The best way to resist temptation is to avoid exposure to it.

The same is true of your bedroom. This should be for sleep and for sex, nothing else. If you have a TV in the bedroom, or you take your mobile phone to bed with you, the temptation will be to use them, and that can be highly disruptive.

There's a widespread myth that light coming from your computer or mobile phone (blue light) is bad for you because it switches off production of the sleep hormone, melatonin. In reality, light levels produced by these devices are too low to do much damage and the real reason they are disruptive is because they are exciting your brain just when you want it to be nice and relaxed. I always put my mobile on sleep mode and try to avoid looking at it in the hour leading up to bedtime. Anyone who has kids will know just how disruptive social media can be. We had regular battles with our kids about not having laptops and mobile phones in the bedroom when they were teenagers, but we felt it was a fight we had to win. Which we did. Mostly.

Sleep deprivation is spectacularly bad for teen brains and the whole point of social media is that it has been designed by evil geniuses with the sole purpose of keeping you hooked.

Again, it's like food. The reason we find foods like chocolate and crisps so hard to resist is that they have been created and manufactured to be moreish. When I start on a bar of chocolate, I have to eat the whole thing. It's just as well I have never got to grips with Facebook or Instagram.

8pm: your wind-down routine

If you go to bed with your head buzzing and your guts still trying to digest the snack you just ate, you will find it harder to go to sleep. A proper wind-down routine begins several hours before you go to bed.

STOP EATING

Ideally, you will have finished your last meal of the day at least three hours before you go to bed. That is what I was recently advised by Dr Satchin Panda, a professor at the Salk Institute in the US and a world expert in chronobiology and circadian clock research. He is the scientist behind a form of intermittent fasting called time-restricted eating (TRE), which is practised by numerous celebrities, such as Hugh Jackman and Miranda Kerr, as well as some of the major techies in Silicon Valley. Elon Musk does it, as does Geoffrey Woo, the CEO of HVMN, a 'human enhancement' company.

The idea behind TRE is that limiting the window within which you eat will help you lose weight, improve your cholesterol and blood sugar levels, make you sharper and help you sleep better.

In one form of TRE, 16:8, you might stop eating at 8pm and not eat again until midday the next day. It is called 16:8 because you go 16 hours without eating and eat all your meals within an eight-hour window.

Dr Panda told me that he thinks most people will find 14:10 easier to stick to, and that is what he aims for himself. He has an evening meal with his family around 6pm and then doesn't eat again until 8am the next morning.

Why does he think it is so important to stop eating several hours before bed? Well, it is mainly to do with your core body temperature. Your body temperature naturally starts to fall as bedtime approaches, driven by your circadian clock. This fall also helps trigger sleep. The trouble with late-night eating is it raises body temperature. When a late-night snack hits your stomach, your gut has to spring into action to break down and absorb the food you've just eaten. This increase in gut activity means your core body temperature will remain high, just when you want it to go down.

> **But I like to have a nice milky drink, or a bowl of cereal, just before going to bed!**
>
> Drinking cocoa or having a bowl of cereal just before bed may be soothing but it's a bad idea. Your pancreas (which produces insulin) needs downtime and, driven by your circadian clock, will have closed down for the night. So it won't be ready for the big sugar hit that cereal or cocoa will deliver. This sugar hit will cause your blood sugars to rise and keep on rising into the night, which

is bad for sleep as well as for your body. Any fat you eat in your snack will also cause levels of fat in your blood to rise further and faster than they would earlier in the day and take longer to come down.

A few years ago, I did an experiment on myself in which I ate exactly the same high-fat, high-carb meal at 10am and 10pm. Whereas my fat and blood sugar levels rose and fell quite quickly after the morning meal, in the evening they were both still rising well after midnight.

Another reason to avoid a late-night snack or glass of milk is that any protein in the food will cause your stomach to release acid. If you suffer from acid reflux, stay away from anything but water in the two hours running up to bedtime.

One of the other major benefits of TRE is that it gives the lining of your gut, which takes a fearful bashing during the day, more time to repair itself. It's a bit like trying to repair a motorway; you can't do it while cars are driving up and down in the day, so you have to wait till night-time to close it down. If you don't give your gut time to repair, you may develop a condition called leaky gut syndrome, which occurs when bacteria that are living in your guts escape through the damaged stomach lining into your bloodstream, causing inflammation, bloating and pain.

But what if you feel hungry? Dr Panda told me that once you get used to his regime you no longer get late-night munchies. In fact, you will find, after a couple of weeks, that if you do have a late-night snack it will leave you feeling uncomfortably bloated.

ALCOHOL: A MIXED BLESSING

Alcohol is a tricky one. Almost everything I've read says that you shouldn't drink alcohol at night because, while it may help you drop off, it will lead to snoring and more fragmented sleep later on. Although that may be true for heavy drinkers, there is some evidence that points to potential benefits for light drinkers.

A couple of years ago, Israeli scientists recruited 224 teetotal diabetics[47] and randomly allocated them to drinking a medium-sized glass (150ml) of either red wine, white wine or mineral water with their evening meal, every evening, for two years. The wine and water were provided free of charge and the empty bottles collected afterwards to make sure they really were drinking regularly.

So what happened? Well, red-wine drinkers will be delighted to hear it was the group drinking red wine who came out on top. Not only were there significant improvements in their cholesterol and blood sugar levels, but they also reported better-quality sleep.

In another more recent study,[48] this time carried out by an American team, researchers found that exposing mice to small amounts of alcohol, equivalent to a human drinking a glass of wine, made their glymphatic systems (the channels in your brain that open up in deep sleep) more efficient at washing out the brain and removing waste.

What makes this study particularly intriguing is that the woman behind it, Dr Maiken Nedergaard, is also the scientist who first revealed the existence of the glymphatic system in 2012. As she points out, 'Studies have shown that while heavy drinking for many years leads to an increased risk of cognitive decline, low-to-moderate alcohol intake is associated with a lower risk of dementia. This study may help explain why.'

I personally find that one glass of red wine with dinner has little effect on my sleep, but a couple of glasses makes it measurably worse. If you drink every night and suffer from insomnia, do try giving up drinking for a week and see what happens. I recently met a woman at a party who said she used to drink half a bottle of wine every night and thought it was helping her sleep. But when she gave up drinking for a week (because she was taking antibiotics), she quickly noticed how much better she felt. 'After years of waking up almost every night and fretting, now I almost always sleep through the night and I feel fantastic. I have so much energy. I still drink on special occasions but giving up routine drinking has changed my life.'

9.30pm: find something soothing to do

DIM THE LIGHTS

By 9.30pm, your pineal gland should be busy pumping out the hormone melatonin, which in turn will be orchestrating the rest of your brain, getting it lined up for a night of sleep. Melatonin levels typically start to rise about 9pm and peak in the early hours of the morning.

Really bright light switches off the production of melatonin, particularly light in the blue frequency. That's why mobile phone manufacturers now sell products that reduce the amount of blue light they emit at night. But, as I've said before, this is a bit of a con.

The problem with mobile phones and tablets is not so much the light they produce, but the fact that they stimulate the brain just when you need to slow down.

Ideally, you should switch off the bright lights in your house and go for more subdued lighting. Tim Peake, the British astronaut who spent six months on the International Space Station, told me they have recently altered the lighting on the space station so it gradually changes, over the course of a 'day', from light that is more in the blue frequency first thing, to light that is more in the red frequency as the 'day' progresses, mimicking the light changes that happen back on Earth.

The Hadza, hunter-gatherers who live in Tanzania, shun artificial lighting and have no word for 'insomnia'. They gather around the campfire at night, to share stories and experiences, before heading to bed a few hours after the sun has set.

HAVE A WARM BATH

Instead of relaxing by knocking back a few drinks, you would be better off having a warm bath (with a few drops of an essential oil, such as lavender), reading a book or listening to music. Studies have shown that having a warm bath or shower an hour before bedtime can help you fall asleep and stay asleep.[49]

But for it to have an effect you probably have to be in the bath for at least 10 minutes and it has to be at least an hour before bedtime. Why? Well, not surprisingly, getting into a hot bath will heat you up. It will also increase the circulation of blood to your skin, hands and feet. When you get out of the bath, after a good, long soak, and don your kimono, your body will continue to radiate heat. In time this will cool your core temperature down. The critical words are 'in time'. This whole cycle of heating and cooling takes about an hour. Simply dashing into the shower for a couple of minutes just before jumping into bed (which is what I tend to do most nights) isn't going to make you sleepy.

LISTEN TO MUSIC

According to the National Sleep Foundation,[50] studies have shown that older adults who listen to relaxing music before bed fall asleep faster, sleep longer, wake up less during the night and rate their nights as more restful. Apparently, slow tunes with a rhythm of 60 to 80 beats per minute, which you're likely to find in classical, jazz or folk music, are the most effective sleep inducers.

10.30pm: countdown to sleep

TRY KEEPING A 'TO-DO' JOURNAL

As well as keeping a sleep diary (to be filled in every morning), you might, as part of your final wind-down to sleep, try keeping a 'to-do' journal. The idea is that you write down a list of the things you need to do the next day. This will, hopefully, mean you spend less time agonising about your to-do list in the middle of the night.

Does this work? Yes, there is evidence that it does. A small study of American university[51] students found that those who spent five minutes writing about the day ahead went to sleep an average of nine minutes faster. Nine minutes doesn't sound a lot, but it is similar to the impact of taking a sleeping pill. Keeping a journal also reduced the tendency to wake up in the night.

While you've got your journal out, you might also want to write in it three good things that happened to you that day. It can be anything from a friend admiring your clothes to watching a great sunset. Expressing gratitude, also known as 'counting your blessings', is a proven way to reduce stress, one of the main causes of insomnia.

When I was young, I was quite religious and I used to kneel by my bed most evenings and pray. I would thank God for the good things that had happened and ask him to forgive me for the stupid and thoughtless things I had done. It was a good way of finding peace before getting into bed. I'm no longer a believer but I find the practice of writing down three good things has a similar effect.

Thinking of, and then, importantly, writing down three good things works because it shifts your thoughts towards the pleasant things that happened during the day, helping to counter the natural tendency at night to ruminate and worry – it is these ruminations that frequently keep us awake.

CONSIDER TAKING MELATONIN

There are dangers to taking sleeping pills, at least in the long term (for more information on sleeping pills and sleep remedies, see the Q&A on page 126). I take the occasional sleeping pill, such as zopiclone, when I travel long distance. It really helps me sleep on the plane and also combat jet lag when I land (see Chapter 3). I don't use it otherwise.

Melatonin is different. As I explained earlier, it is a hormone that is produced by the pineal gland, a pea-shaped structure in the middle of your brain. It is connected to your brain clock, the suprachiasmatic nucleus (SCN). When it gets dark, your SCN tells your pineal gland to start releasing melatonin. Rising levels of melatonin help coordinate the other parts of your brain that tip you into sleep. Levels peak at around 3am and then decline.

Synthetic melatonin is widely available and can be quite effective. So who should take it and when? As we get older, our brains tend to produce less melatonin, which could be why our sleep deteriorates. That is also why melatonin works best in people over the age of 55.

In the UK, Australia and most of Europe, you can only get melatonin on prescription, whereas in the US you can pick it up at any chemist. I normally buy a few bottles when I am in the US, or order them online from a reputable American company like iherb. It is perfectly legal to buy melatonin this way, but it is illegal to sell it on.

In the US, controlled-release melatonin is the recommended first-line treatment for older adults with insomnia. It has very few side effects (I have never noticed any); in fact, in one study[52] there were fewer side effects in those taking melatonin than in those taking placebo pills.

An Australian government report from 2011[53] concluded that taking 2mg of melatonin, one to two hours before bedtime, was safe and effective for people over the age of 55. They said it was safe to consume it daily for up to 13 weeks and that, unlike sleeping pills, there was no evidence that you get rebound insomnia when you stop. Taking it every night for months on end may not be a great idea because in a study in which people took melatonin or a placebo every day for six months, the researchers found that by six months there was not much difference between the two groups.[54]

Though it appears to be safe, the Australian government report suggested it should not be used by children, pregnant women or those with liver problems.

Although you are supposed to take it an hour or so before going to bed, I prefer taking it at 3am, when I wake up and find it hard to get back to sleep. Since melatonin has a half-life of 3–4.5 hours, this should make me dopey the next morning, but it doesn't.

I take 2mg, slow release, but if that doesn't work you could try experimenting with higher doses (up to 5mg is safe). Unless I'm jet-lagged, I take melatonin no more than once or twice a week.

Q&A

Why can't I just take some sleeping pills?
By sleeping pills, most people mean benzodiazepines, such as temazepam and the Z drugs, such as zopiclone. These can be helpful in the very short term for treating acute anxiety or distress of the sort that

follows a bereavement or job loss. And I use zopiclone to help with jet lag. But like all medications, they have potential side effects and they become less effective over time.

If I start taking them, will I become addicted?

Modern sleeping pills are less addictive than the old-fashioned barbiturates, but they can become habit-forming quite rapidly. That is why a GP will rarely give repeat prescriptions, saving them for short-term use. If a patient is going through a more prolonged period of stress, affecting their sleep, then a GP might prescribe a low dose of amitriptyline – a drug used at higher doses for anxiety and depression, but which can improve sleep at a lower dose. It leaves some people feeling a bit dopey or 'hung over' first thing in the morning and it can have irritating side effects such as a dry mouth. It can also interact with other medications.

What about over-the-counter remedies?

There are a whole range of over-the-counter supplements and herbal remedies that probably help a bit if you have a short-term problem, but they don't offer a long-term solution because they do not tackle the underlying causes of insomnia. If you are taking other medications, you should consult your doctor as many of them will interact with other drugs. Also be very careful what you take if you are pregnant or breastfeeding.

Chlorphenamine, also known by the brand name Piriton, is a popular over-the-counter antihistamine used to treat hay fever and insect bites and sometimes as a sleep remedy as it makes you feel drowsy. In rare cases it can cause allergic responses and may interact with other drugs, particularly some antidepressants.

Diphenhydramine, another sleep-inducing antihistamine, is found in products such as Benadryl. Like chlorphenamine, it seems to be reasonably effective and has similar potential side effects.

A few small studies suggest that taking magnesium supplements may help elderly people fall asleep faster. On the whole you would be better off boosting your magnesium levels by eating foods that are rich in magnesium, such as avocados, leafy green veg, legumes and nuts, like cashews and almonds.

Tryptophan can be taken in moderate doses as a supplement to improve sleep, but it has been found in some cases to interact with other medicines such as antidepressants. It can also cause side effects such as sweating, anxiety, nausea and vomiting.

Valerian is a commonly used sleep-promoting herbal supplement. There have been studies in which people taking 300–900mg of valerian before bedtime found it improved self-rated sleep quality, but I could find no long-term studies. Again, watch out for drug interactions.

What about essential oils?

The most popular ones for helping you drift off are lavender, vanilla, rose and bergamot (a type of orange). You can put a few drops in a warm bath, or you may prefer to scent the air with a diffuser or spray. If you want to make your own, add 4–5 drops of essential oil to half a cup of water and then pour it into an empty scent bottle. You can also put a couple of drops on the underside of a pillow or on the sheet but do not apply directly to the skin as these oils are highly concentrated and can cause irritation. Do they make a difference? I found one review article[55] which concluded that they might help with mild sleep disturbances.

Lavender is the most widely studied. At the very least they will make your bedroom smell delightful and refocus your thoughts on experiencing the lovely scent rather than on your worries.

The long night of the soul

Let's assume that you follow my advice and go to bed at 11pm, after having a lovely pre-bed routine, then quickly fall asleep and wake up feeling refreshed and thinking: 'I must recommend this book to other people.'

But what if you don't? What if you are still lying there, staring at the ceiling, listening to your partner snoring away, worrying about not going to sleep and besieged by negative thoughts?

You could try doing some breathing exercises or using cognitive behavioural techniques to help you challenge your thoughts (see page 132). On the other hand, it could be that when you went to bed you just weren't sleepy enough.

The rule of thumb is that if you feel like you haven't fallen asleep within 20 minutes of closing your eyes then you should get out of bed and out of your bedroom. (I say 'feel like' because I don't want you to be constantly checking the clock. It is better to just guess how much time has gone by.)

The technical term for this process is 'stimulus control' and the reason you need to get up rather than just lie there is that you must associate bed with sleep and sex, nothing else. If you lie awake in bed, night after night, wrestling with your mental demons, this will trigger all sorts of unhelpful associations in your brain and body.

We have known, ever since the Russian physiologist Ivan Pavlov first demonstrated that he could make dogs salivate at the sound of a bell, how easy it is to create powerful, unconscious links. You do not want to reinforce, consciously or unconsciously, any associations between 'going to bed' and 'not being able to fall asleep'. So if you can't go to sleep within what feels like 20 minutes, get out of your nice warm bed and head for another room, where you will sit and while away the time until you start to feel sleepy. This is not an excuse to go back on the laptop, catch up with a rerun of *Friends* or check out Facebook. If you are going to try melatonin, this may be a good time to do it. It will take about 30 minutes to kick in.

Ideally, you'll spend this time listening to soothing music or a dull podcast, or reading a book you have read before. I never have any difficulty falling asleep, but I often wake up in the middle of the night. Sometimes I am able to go back to sleep, sometimes not. I have a pile of books downstairs that I have read many times and which I work my way through as I wait for my sleep drive to reassert itself.

NIGHT-TIME BREATHING EXERCISES TO REDUCE STRESS AND PAIN

Yogic breathing (pranayama) is a form of controlled breathing that has been practised for thousands of years. It is often done in conjunction with meditation or yoga. It reduces stress by activating the parasympathetic system, part of your autonomic nervous system. Activating the parasympathetic system causes your heart to slow and your blood pressure to drop. When I am struggling to sleep, the first thing I attempt is deep breathing, also known as belly breathing. In everyday life we tend to take shallow breaths, so this may feel a bit weird to start with.

You start by taking a slow, deep inhale through the nose, allowing the air to really fill your lungs. Put a hand on your belly – you should feel it inflate. Hold it for a count of two, then breathe out slowly through your mouth. The first few times you do it, it will feel unnatural, so you need to practise during the daytime. You will notice that as you do this, your heart rate will slow and you will start to feel more relaxed.

There are lots of different breathing techniques. The one I favour is 4-2-4.

- Breathe in deeply through your nose while mentally counting to 4.
- Hold your breath to a count of 2.
- Breathe out through your mouth to a count of 4.
- Try doing this for a couple of minutes. It should feel really relaxing.

You'll find more on breathing techniques on page 207.

CHALLENGING YOUR THOUGHTS

Many people report that they are kept awake by crazy thoughts that seem to surface in the middle of the night. These could be anything from worrying about their kids to fretting about the damage that not sleeping is having on their brain. One way of dealing with these thoughts is to get out of bed and do something distracting, rather than engage with them. But you could also try a bit of Cognitive Behavioural Therapy (CBT). It is an approach that teaches you to challenge those thoughts. Although they are generated inside your brain, your thoughts are not real and they can be challenged in the same way you might argue with your dad when he says something particularly annoying.

Examples of the sort of thoughts you can be taught to challenge include:

'I won't get to sleep and if I don't then I will feel really tired tomorrow and won't be able to function.'

Challenge: 'I'm sure I will get to sleep, I normally do. But even if I don't, it will be fine. One bad night's sleep is OK.'

'It's the same every single night, I just lie here worrying. Why can't I ever get a good night's sleep?'

Challenge: 'That isn't true, it doesn't happen every night. Yes, it's annoying, but it will pass.'

Since negative thoughts like these are often part of a lifelong pattern of thinking, successfully challenging them is rarely easy. That's why, if you want to learn how to do it effectively, you may need to see a qualified therapist.

3.30am and wide awake?

Although some people find it hard to go to sleep, the most common sleep problem is waking up in the middle of the night. It is often because you need to go to the loo, and once you have woken up it is hard to get back to sleep.

It typically happens four or five hours after you have fallen asleep, when you have been through three 90-minute sleep cycles and are in the light stage of the sleep cycle. To use my diving analogy, it's as if you have come to the surface for a swift gulp of air but find you can't then get back down to the deep again.

What should you do? Essentially, my advice is do the same as you do when you can't get to sleep in the first place: try deep breathing, try challenging your negative thoughts, and if, within 20 minutes, none of that is working, get out of bed.

The main thing is to try not to worry about the fact that you are awake when you would much rather be asleep, or what this means for the following day. Going down that road will just make things much, much worse.

I find it useful to reflect on the fact that waking up in the middle of the night is a natural thing and that it used to be seen as totally normal before we decided that we had to sleep through the night, as I explained on page 58.

Some people use this period of wakefulness as an opportunity to enjoy a bit of night life. I was recently contacted by someone who likes to go out and do some photography at 3am, before heading back to bed and a second sleep. Others find 3am is a good time to write. Charles Dickens would frequently wander the streets of London at 3am, and even wrote a book about it, *Night Walks*. These strolls (which lasted up to five hours) gave him powerful insights into poverty, vice and drunkenness, which he used in his novels. As dawn approached, Dickens would often go to a local railway station to watch the morning mail arrive. 'The station lamps would burst out ablaze,' he wrote. 'The porters would emerge, the cabs and trucks would rattle to their places, and, finally, the bell would strike up, and the train would come banging in, knowing that sunrise was not too far away.'

He would then head home, to bed.

EXTREME LARKINESS

If you are an extreme lark, you might just choose to get up and stay up.

The American actor Mark Wahlberg likes to rise at 2:30am. He starts his day with prayers, followed by breakfast and then a workout. I know this because he often posts on Instagram under the hashtag #4amclub. His daily schedule looks something like this:

2.30am	Wake up
2.45am	Prayers and then breakfast
3.40am	First workout of the day
1.00pm	Lunch
4.00pm	Second workout of the day
5.00pm	Shower
5.30pm	Dinner
7.30pm	Off to bed

Tim Cook, head of Apple, the most valuable company in the world, is also an early riser.[56] He gets up at 3.45am, does his emails for an hour and then heads to the gym before putting in a full working day. However bad my insomnia has become, I have never been tempted to do this.

Time to get up and embrace the day

Assuming you are not a teenager or an extreme lark, then 7am is a typical time to get up. Although some over-achievers get up much earlier, others like Elon Musk (up at 7am), Amazon founder Jeff Bezos (7am to 8am) and Mark Zuckerberg, head of Facebook (up by 8am) seem to have more normal sleep patterns.[57]

DO A BRIEF WORKOUT

The one thing that all these top execs do is exercise as soon as they get up in the morning. I try to emulate them. When I roll out of bed, the first thing I do most mornings is a series of resistance exercises, which include press-ups and squats (see page 199). My routine normally takes less than five minutes. I have to do them straight away or I know I will never get around to doing them.

Unlike aerobic exercise (running, swimming, walking), resistance exercise is particularly good at building and preserving muscles. Doing resistance exercises is also a great way of improving the quality of your sleep. A recent review article in the journal *Sleep*[57] concluded that 'resistance exercise improves all aspects of sleep, with the greatest benefit for sleep quality … In addition to the sleep benefits, resistance exercise training improves anxiety and depression.'

The great thing about my regime is I don't need to go to the gym and it doesn't cost me anything. Plus it is over really fast.

LIGHT EXPOSURE THERAPY

When I have the time, I take our dog for a 30-minute walk before breakfast. Part of the reason for doing this is to get the exercise, but mainly it is to expose myself to lots of early-morning light.

The amount of light you experience in your house, or in the car on the way to work, is only a fraction of what you get when you are outdoors, even when it is overcast and gloomy. The point of going out into the early-morning light is that it will reset your internal clock, and let your body know that the day has begun.

During the long, dark winter, or if you really struggle with getting up in the morning, you might want to invest in a light box. A good one produces 10,000 lux (a measure of light intensity), which is similar to the levels you get outdoors on a bright spring morning. Light levels in your house or at the office are more likely to be a miserable 25 to 50 lux.

The great thing about light boxes is that you can work at your computer or read a book with one on a table beside you.

> **Light boxes and SAD**
>
> I first came across light boxes when I was making a film about SAD (Seasonal Affective Disorder), also known as the winter blues. People who suffer from SAD start feeling uncharacter- istically low at the start of winter and perk up again in the spring. Many of us experience the winter blues to some degree,

but around 5% of the population find the winter months truly crippling. Typical symptoms include low mood, feeling sleepy during the day (despite lots of sleep) and having a mad craving for carbs. To treat SAD, you need to use a light box for at least 30 minutes every morning. A light box is also a good way to help turn an owl into a lark because it can help reset your internal clock. But a warning: when you use your light box depends on what your sleep problem is. If you are a super-lark, waking up much earlier than you want (something which is common as people get older) and you are struggling to stay awake at night, then you should not use a light box in the morning.

In fact, you might want to shun the early morning light as much as possible. Instead, you should aim to get a good blast of light in the late afternoon, thereby delaying the release of melatonin.

WHAT ABOUT BREAKFAST?

As we all know, Breakfast Is the Most Important Meal of the Day. What you may not know is that the slogan first appeared in 1917 in a magazine called *Good Health* – a magazine that, surprise, surprise, was edited by none other than Dr John Harvey Kellogg, one of the creators of Kellogg's cornflakes.

Although it is a slogan that has been endlessly repeated, there is no scientific consensus about the value of eating breakfast first thing in the morning. A recent meta-analysis published in the *British Medical*

Journal,[59] which looked at evidence from 13 breakfast studies, concluded that telling adults that eating breakfast will help them lose weight is unwise because 'it could have the opposite effect'.

One advantage of breaking your fast later in the day is that it extends your overnight fast, giving your body more time to get on with essential repairs.

IS IT OK TO HAVE AN AFTERNOON NAP?

Naps used to be a very Mediterranean thing to do. When I travelled around Greece and Spain in the 1970s, people would often head home in the early afternoon for a brief siesta. That way of life has largely gone.

The siesta was rebranded as the 'power nap' in the early 2000s by James Maas, a former Cornell psychology professor turned corporate sleep guru. He claimed that a 15- to 20-minute snooze in the early afternoon was all you needed to recharge your body and brain.

There is something to this, though when and how long you nap is critical. Ideally, you should take your nap seven hours after you wake up (so if you woke at 6.30am your nap should be around 1.30pm).

Your nap needs to be long enough to be refreshing, but not so long that you sink into a deep sleep. If that happens, you run the risk of sleep inertia: not only waking up feeling groggy and even drowsier than you did before, but also finding it harder to go to sleep that evening. Though you can nap in a chair, it would be more effective to nap on a bed in a nice quiet room while wearing a face mask to block out the lights. Some employers, like Google, provide sleep pods for employees. Shift workers benefit most from having naps, as discussed in Chapter 3.

Do remember to set your alarm because you really don't want to sleep the afternoon away.

FINALLY, DINNER …

And so we come full circle. If you want to try TRE, you might want to nudge your evening meal earlier so you finish eating by 8pm at the latest. That's what we aim to do in the Mosley household.

You may also want to try some of the delicious sleep-enhancing recipes that Clare has created – you'll find them at the end of the book. In the next chapter, I am going to explain why some foods are so much better at helping you sleep than others.

Summary

If you want to improve your sleep, you must first create a sleep window, the time at which you plan to go to bed and get up each morning, and stick to it as rigidly as you can.

- Improve your sleep hygiene by fostering good bedtime habits, limiting caffeine and alcohol, clearing electronic gadgets from your bedroom, and ensuring it is cool, dark and quiet.
- Unlike sleeping pills, melatonin seems to improve sleep quality without causing addiction. There is limited evidence for the effectiveness of magnesium, lavender or other over-the-counter remedies.
- Breathing exercises are an excellent way of slowing your heart and distracting your thoughts.

- If you wake in the night and find it hard to get back to sleep, get out of bed and do not return until you feel sleepy.
- Invest in a light box or go for an early-morning walk or run. Half an hour of outdoor light every morning will help reset your internal clock.
- If you want to take a nap, make sure you do so no later than 2pm and for no longer than 20 minutes.

6. Eating your way to a good night's sleep

As I mentioned in the previous chapter, a few years ago I wrote a book called *The Clever Guts Diet*, about the impact that the food we eat has on our microbiome, the trillions of microbes that live in our guts. The book included recipes and advice, shown to boost the good bacteria and minimise the bad. Improving your microbiome can help you lose weight, boost your immune system and improve your mood. Since I wrote that book, there has been lots more research into the impact of food on mood, including some that has looked at the effect that specific foods have on our sleep. For example:

- An experiment carried out by researchers from the Institute of Human Nutrition in New York[60] showed for the first time that feeding volunteers a diet rich in fibre and protein led to more deep sleep, while getting the same volunteers to eat foods rich in sugar and simple carbs led to more fragmented sleep.

- Another study, from the same group,[61] which looked at the diet and sleeping patterns of more than 2200 people across America, found that those with a high M score (see page 145) slept longer and better than those eating a more typical American diet.
- A study published in 2017,[62] carried out by Professor Felice Jacka, director of the Food & Mood Centre in Melbourne, Australia, showed for the first time that putting people with moderate to severe depression on a Med-style diet led to such big improvements in mood that many were no longer clinically depressed.
- In a more recent study, published in October 2019,[63] researchers from the US showed that people who have higher levels of certain microbes in their guts, particularly those from the phylum Bacteroidetes, enjoy deeper, more efficient sleep and less waking at night than those with lower levels.

I will go into these and many other studies in more detail later on in this chapter, but first let's lay to rest some commonly accepted ideas about sleep-friendly foods.

A load of old turkey

The idea that certain foods can aid sleep is not a new one. But you might be surprised to learn which really do impact sleep. They're not the ones that are commonly talked about.

There is, for example, a widespread myth that eating turkey makes you sleepy. According to a self-styled sleep expert I found on the internet, 'Turkey is rich in an amino acid called tryptophan, which goes to your brain and is converted to serotonin, which helps you sleep.'

In fact, turkey contains no more tryptophan than chicken or beef, and a lot less than nuts, seeds or cheese. Another problem with this claim is that although eating lots of turkey will raise the levels of tryptophan in your blood, it has no effect on the levels in your brain because so little of it crosses the blood–brain barrier. For this reason, taking tryptophan capsules is also a waste of time.

Two other foods that I've seen hailed as sleep enhancers are tart cherries and kiwi fruit.

Claims about the benefits of tart cherries are based on a couple of small studies done in elderly people with insomnia who drank a large glass of cherry juice (240ml), twice a day for two weeks.[64] There were some modest changes in sleep quality but the notion that it works because 'tart cherries contain melatonin' is clearly nonsense. You would need to drink about 500 litres a day to get a big enough dose of melatonin to make a difference.

And as for kiwi fruit, well, there was one small study from Singapore[65] in which the researchers asked 24 volunteers to eat two kiwi fruits an hour before bedtime, every night for four weeks. The study found that it made a small difference, but when I tried following this regime it made my sleep, if anything, worse. It also put me off kiwi fruit for a long time.

Another popular myth is that eating cheese gives you bad dreams. Eating anything that is rich in saturated fat just before you go to bed is likely to disrupt your sleep, but there's no evidence that cheese is worse than any other food, or that it triggers nightmares. The claim that cheese causes nightmares seems to have started with Charles Dickens's book, *A Christmas Carol*, in which the central character, Ebenezer Scrooge, blames his disturbing visions on eating cheese. But when, in 2005, researchers from Surrey University asked 200 men to eat different cheeses every night for a week and record their dreams, they found no evidence that eating cheese induced nightmares, though it may have resulted in more vivid dreams.[66]

So which foods do improve the quality of your sleep?

Let's start with my favourite way of eating, the Mediterranean diet, the traditional diet of the countries that border the Mediterranean Sea. I have been a huge fan ever since I discovered that it is not only super-tasty but also has a wide range of health benefits. Studies[67] have shown that eating a Mediterranean diet will:

- Cut your risk of having a heart attack or stroke by around 30%;
- Cut your risk of developing type 2 diabetes by 50%;
- Cut your risk of developing breast cancer by up to 70%.

The traditional Mediterranean diet involves consuming lots of olive oil, nuts, oily fish, fruit, veg and wholegrains. You also eat reasonable amounts of full-fat yoghurt and cheese, as well as a glass or two of red wine with the evening meal. There is not much room in this diet for cakes, biscuits or highly processed food. You can calculate how 'Mediterranean' your current diet is with the following simple quiz.

What is your M score?

Add a point for each 'yes' answer. A score of 10 or higher is good.

1. Do you use olive oil as your main cooking fat and dressing?
2. Do you eat two or more portions of vegetables a day? (1 serving = 200g/7oz)
3. Do you eat two or more portions of fruit a day? (No points for sweet tropical fruits)
4. Do you eat less than one serving of processed meat a day? (1 serving = 100g/3.5oz)
5. Do you eat full-fat yoghurt at least three times a week?
6. Do you eat three or more servings of legumes – e.g. peas, beans, lentils – a week? (1 serving = 150g/5.25oz)
7. Do you eat three or more servings of wholegrains a week? (1 serving = 150g/5.25oz)
8. Do you eat oily fish, prawns or shellfish three or more times a week? (100–150g/3.5–5.25oz fish)
9. Do you eat sweet treats like cakes, biscuits, etc., fewer than three times a week?
10. Do you eat a serving of nuts (30g/1oz) three or more times a week?
11. Do you cook with garlic, onions and tomatoes at least three times a week?

12. Do you average around seven glasses of wine a week?

13. Do you sit at the table to eat at least twice a day?

14. Do you drink sweet, fizzy beverages less than once a week?

Notes:

- Potatoes do not count as a vegetable.
- Sweet tropical fruits include melon, grapes, pineapple and bananas.
- Processed meat includes ham, bacon, sausages and salami.
- Whole grains include quinoa, whole rye, bulgur wheat.
- Nuts include walnuts, almonds, cashew nuts and peanuts and should be unsalted.
- Drinking much more than seven units of alcohol a week can be harmful.

SCORE : ⬜ /14

The Mediterranean diet and sleep

Although most of the research looking at the Mediterranean diet has focused on its impact on reducing heart disease, cancer, dementia and diabetes, in the last couple of years there have been a couple of big studies published in reputable journals, looking at its effect on sleep.

In May 2019, for example, a study in Italy[68] looked at the link between what Italian adults are eating and how well they are sleeping. For the MEAL study,[69] researchers collected data from 1314 men and women living in Catania, one of the largest cities on the island of Sicily.

The researchers took detailed records of what the participants ate and then used the results of their completed food questionnaires to divide them into four groups, based on their M score, ranging from low to high Mediterranean diet adherence.

The participants also filled in the Pittsburgh sleep quality index, a more detailed version of the quiz I mentioned on page 89.

When the researchers compared what they ate with how well they slept, they found that those with a high M score were more than twice as likely to enjoy decent-quality sleep as those with a low M score. They not only slept longer, but they had a higher sleep efficiency and were less likely to have a disturbed night.

Interestingly, this was true only for those who were a healthy weight, or a bit overweight. The men and women who were obese (with a BMI over 30) were not protected from poor sleep by a healthy diet.

These findings were replicated by another big study[70] that looked at the links between diet and sleep in more than 2000 middle-aged men

and women in the US. Again, there was a clear link between participants' M score and how well they slept.

The problem with observational studies, like the two I've just
described, is that you can never be entirely sure of the extent to which
it is a good diet that leads to better sleep, or vice versa. As I pointed
out earlier, when people are sleep deprived they tend to eat more
junk food.

That's why I was pleased to come across a novel intervention study
conducted at Cornell University in New York,[71] in which the researchers manipulated the subjects' diet and then saw what effect that had
on their sleep.

For this study, they asked 26 adults – 13 men and 13 women – to
spend five nights in a sleep lab, wired up to machines so their sleep could
be monitored in detail. During this time, the participants ate meals
that contained varying amounts of fat, protein, carbs, fibre and sugar.

It turned out that when they ate meals containing more saturated
fat, carbs and sugar, they had lighter, more disrupted sleep. But when
they ate meals that were richer in protein and fibre, they got to sleep
faster and spent more time in deep sleep.

There are a number of reasons why eating a Med diet helps sleep.
These include the fact that:

1. The foods in this diet, like olive oil, oily fish, legumes and
   vegetables, contain anti-inflammatory compounds, such as oleic
   acid, omega-3 fatty acids and polyphenols. We know that inflammation leads to arthritis and other painful conditions that keep
   people awake at night. We also know that neuroinflammation

(inflammation of the brain), which becomes more common as we get older, contributes to poor sleep and dementia.

2. Going on a Mediterranean diet boosts levels of the 'good' bacteria in your gut – these in turn can produce powerful anti-inflammatory agents, as well as 'feel good' chemicals which reduce anxiety. Since one of the main reasons people stay awake at night is because they are ruminating and fretting, anything that improves mood is likely to be good for sleep.

The impact of the Mediterranean diet on mood

I am a big fan of Professor Felice Jacka, the dynamic director of the Food & Mood Centre at Deakin University in Melbourne, Australia, and the pioneering studies that she and her colleagues are doing, showing how the foods we eat influence our brain, mood and mental health.

I came across her work in 2017, when she published the results of the SMILES trial.[72] It was the first intervention study looking at whether putting people on a healthier diet could improve depression. It was truly ground-breaking, and because it was so revolutionary it was also hard to get off the ground.

In retrospect, it is astonishing that it took scientists such a long time to run an experiment like this one. Felice had initially wanted to recruit 180 people with moderate to severe depression for the SMILES trial, but after three long, hard years of trying, she and her team had only managed to recruit 67.

The problem with having modest numbers of people in a study is that it is much harder to prove that your intervention has made a difference. Felice realised that the impact of the diet would have to be pretty dramatic for any results to be deemed 'significant'.

Once they'd recruited their 67 subjects, her team randomly allocated 33 of them to a dietician who helped them start eating what they called a 'ModiMed diet', while the other 34 got 'social support'.

Those allocated to the ModiMed diet were encouraged to eat more wholegrains, vegetables, fruit, legumes and unsalted nuts, as well as some eggs and dairy. They were also asked to eat three tablespoons of olive oil a day, and fish and chicken at least twice a week. Perhaps surprisingly, they were also advised to eat a moderate amount of lean red meat, such as beef or lamb, three or four times a week. This was because research conducted by Felice and others had shown a link between eating red meat and mood, possibly because of the iron and vitamin B12 content.[73]

The participants were also asked to eat fewer unhealthy foods, such as sweets, refined cereals, fried food, fast food, processed meats and sugary drinks.

After all that preparation – the struggle to recruit volunteers and the meticulous preparation of the diet – Felice told me she was worried that they wouldn't find anything, so she was thrilled when the final results were clearer than she had dared hope.

Just under a third of the people who were put on the ModiMed diet had such large improvements in mood that they were no longer classified as 'depressed'. This was four times better than those getting social support. There was also a significant improvement in the anxiety scores among the ModiMed group. The fact that it was those who made the biggest changes in their diet who saw the greatest improvements strongly suggested that it was the change in diet that had made the difference.

As one of the participants, who had already tried talking therapies and medication, without success, later told the professor: 'The programme was to me a last resort. With its success I am forever grateful.'

Another man, who had suffered from bouts of severe depression, wrote to say that taking part in the study had not only led to big improvements in his mental health, but in his sleep as well.

All of which is impressive and heart-warming, particularly when you appreciate just how hard depression can be to treat with conventional therapies.

What is really encouraging is that other, bigger intervention trials, like the HELFIMED study, have come up with similar findings.[74]

You might be thinking: 'That's fine if you have money, but eating healthily is going to be much more expensive, and therefore not an option for people on a tight budget', but in fact eating healthily can be cheaper than eating badly. The researchers in the SMILES study did a detailed analysis and showed that the cost per person for the diet they are recommending came to A$112 per week. This was far lower than the A$138 per week that the participants were spending, on average, before the experiment.

The key to eating a Med diet cheaply is to go for tinned and frozen foods, which are just as nutritious, as well as fruits and vegetables that are in season. Fibre-rich legumes such as lentils, beans and chickpeas, are a cheap and healthy addition to a meal.

So why did improving their diet have this effect on their mood? Felice thinks it could be because the Med diet reduces inflammation and oxidative stress (the diet contains lots of antioxidants that help mop up free radicals, which otherwise damage brain cells).

But it could also be the diet's effect on the microbiome, which Professor Jacka's team are intensely studying. For more information, I recommend her book, *Brain Changer*.

The microbiome, stress and sleep

You have one to two kilos of microbes, the weight of a large bag of sugar, living in your gut. The 100 trillion microbes that live down there are known as the gut microbiome, and there are as many of them living in your large intestine as there are cells in your body. Which means that you are 50% human and 50% microbe. The human–microbe ratio is so finely balanced that a scientist recently calculated that every time you have a poo (your faeces is 75% dead bacteria), you briefly tip over into becoming more human.[75]

Your gut microbiome consists mainly of bacteria, but there are also fungi, viruses and simple, primitive animals called protozoa down there. In fact, most of us have at least 1000 different species of microbes in our guts, fighting, reproducing and competing. Together they form a wonderfully complicated ecosystem which I like to think of as my gut garden, or internal rainforest. On the whole, we have a good relationship with our microbiome, which is not surprising as we have evolved with it over millions of years. We provide the microbes with a home and they help keep us healthy. We used to think their job was pretty basic: to protect our gut from foreign invaders; to synthesise vitamins like vitamin K, which the body doesn't make; and to produce nasty smells while gobbling up the fibre that our bodies can't digest. Gut gases, better known as farts, are the result of microbe activity.

Now we know the microbiome also:

- Influences our body weight by shaping our appetite and cravings, and deciding how much energy our body extracts from the food we eat. Can your microbiome make you fat? It certainly can.

- Teaches our immune system how to behave. If you don't have the right sort of microbes in your gut, you are at much greater risk of a range of allergic and autoimmune diseases, from asthma to multiple sclerosis.

- Last, but by no means least, it has a big impact on our mood and our sleep, so much so that the study of how the creatures in our guts affect our brains has its own name, 'psychobiotics'.

But how do tiny microbes, who live in your colon, at the far end of your gut, do all these things? Well, they may not have teeth or claws, let alone arms or legs, but they are brilliant chemists. Some of them can take the bits of food our body can't digest (such as fibre) and convert it into hormones that influence our mood – hormones like dopamine, serotonin and GABA (a neurotransmitter that acts in a similar way to the anti-anxiety drug Valium).

Others can turn fibre into a chemical called butyrate, which is brilliant at damping down inflammation. Chronic inflammation is behind a whole range of diseases, including cancer and heart disease. As well as lowering inflammation, butyrate helps to maintain your gut lining, the barrier that keeps bacteria and other toxins from escaping into your blood. The recipes at the back of this book contain foods proven to boost your butyrate levels.

So one of the secrets to a long and healthy life is having a wide range of helpful microbes living in your gut. Like a rainforest, you want your microbiome to be a rich, flourishing population of different creatures.

It's all about diversity

Greater diversity in the gut means having a much more capable and resilient microbial community, one in which there is more competition, so no one species can dominate. It also means hosting lots of different microbes with different chemical talents. We benefit from having firemen-microbes to put out inflammation, builder-microbes to repair the gut wall and pharmo-microbes to make drugs that help us sleep better.

Conversely, we know that having a narrower, less diverse microbiome is associated with a range of chronic diseases, including a higher risk of obesity, inflammation, type 2 diabetes, colorectal cancer and allergies.

Sadly, the microbiome tends to become less diverse as people grow older. This is partly because people tend to eat a narrower range of foods as they get older and partly because they eat more 'convenience' foods, which are highly processed. One of the problems with ultra-processed foods is they often contain emulsifiers, which are added to extend the food's shelf life. Your microbes do not enjoy them.

By the time most people are in their sixties, healthy microbes, like *Lactobacillus* and *Bifidobacterium*, have begun losing ground to pro-inflammatory, opportunistic bacteria. They are called opportunistic because they can cause an infection when given half a chance. Older people also take more prescription drugs, which can play havoc with the microbiome, and they do less exercise, which again reduces microbiome diversity.

There's good evidence that people who manage to keep their gut garden in good shape as they age not only develop less chronic disease but also sleep more soundly.

If you are interested in finding out how diverse your gut garden is and which species are currently living in it, you can have your poo tested. There are lots of different companies, which will sequence your microbiome and provide you with a report of the results for a few hundred dollars.

The process is simple. You can pay for the service on their website and they will send you a plastic tube, a spatula and instructions on how to collect a faecal sample. You put your faeces in the tube, give it a good old shake, stick it in the post and wait for the results. And wait. You can expect the whole thing to take at least two months.

A while ago I sent my faeces off to be tested and the results were certainly interesting. Among other things, they told me that my Simpson index (a measure of just how diverse the biome is) had a score of 7.99. That puts me into the top 30% of 'most diverse microbiomes' of those who have had poo samples tested. Good, though clearly room for improvement.

What is the link between microbial diversity and sleep?

In a study published in October 2019,[76] researchers from Nova Southeastern University in Florida asked a group of men to wear activity monitors and have their sleep patterns analysed over the course of a month. The researchers also collected lots of poo samples from the men, which they then examined closely.

One of the things that came out of this research was clear evidence that the men with the most diverse microbiomes had the best-quality sleep, which included longer total sleep time, higher sleep efficiency and much less night-time waking.

As well as confirming the importance of diversity, researchers identified a number of gut species that were present in higher numbers in the men who slept well. These included Bacteroidetes, which produce GABA, a neurotransmitter that promotes sleep, and *Corynebacterium*, which makes another neurotransmitter, serotonin, which again has been shown to promote sleep.

Another interesting finding was that the men with greater

Black grapes with yoghurt and almonds (p224)

Sweet potato savoury muffins with feta (p228)

Chicken noodles with pak choi (p234)

Curried lentil soup with turmeric (p236)

Dr Tim's hot-smoked salmon salad (p239)

Griddled eggplant with feta and pine nuts (p241)

Prawns and red cabbage slaw on sourdough (p250)

Black bean salad with lime and avocado (p252)

Chicken and veg tray bake (p262)

Meatballs with feta and eggplant (p264)

Mushroom, chickpea and kale curry (p266)

Smokey fish gratin (p270)

Braised red cabbage with walnuts and apple (p277)

Seeded rainbow salad (p279)

Dorset apple cake (p284)

Nutty berry crunch (p287)

microbiome diversity also had higher levels in their blood of interleukin-6, a cytokine that plays an important part in regulating the immune system and influences both sleep and memory.

In an experiment conducted in 2009,[77] German researchers asked a group of healthy young men to spend two nights in their sleep laboratory. Before going to bed each night they were asked to read a short story. Then, the researchers sprayed a fluid containing either interleukin-6 or a harmless placebo into their nostrils. In the morning, the men were asked to write down as many words as they could remember from the story they had read the night before. Inhaling the interleukin-6 clearly made a difference, because not only did they get more deep sleep, compared to the night when they inhaled a placebo, but they could also remember more words from the story.

What all this research suggests is that boosting the good bugs in your microbiome is beneficial for your body and brain, and also has a significant impact on the quality of your sleep. A win-win. So how do you do it? You could start by eating more prebiotics and probiotics.

Prebiotics

A prebiotic is a type of non-digestible plant fibre that acts like a fertiliser to encourage the growth of 'good' bacteria in your gut. Although many veg are rich in fibre, they aren't all classified as prebiotics because many don't contain the sort that will really boost your microbiome. Here are some of the best prebiotics.

BEANS AND LENTILS

Beans and lentils form a big part of the traditional Mediterranean diet. As well as being a great source of prebiotic fibre, they are rich in B vitamins, which have been shown to help sleep, and protein, making them a great alternative to meat. They can be used in soups and stews, with or without meat, and are delicious in curries. Hummus, which you can buy or make yourself from tinned chickpeas, is a nutritious dip, eaten with veggie sticks. Beans and lentils are my top sleep-inducing foods. For ideas on how to enjoy more of them yourself, check out the recipe section on page 223.

ONIONS, LEEKS AND GARLIC

These three members of the Allium family are packed with antioxidants and other nutrients, and are a good source of prebiotic inulin. I love this family of plants and cook with them on a regular basis. Our recipes are full of them. The Spanish make a wonderful tomato base called sofrito, which consists of garlic, onion, paprika and tomatoes all cooked together in olive oil. It's delicious with chicken, fish or prawns.

CHICORY AND RADICCHIO

Chicory and radicchio, vegetables usually eaten in salads, also contain prebiotics. Chicory root is particularly rich in inulin – it accounts for nearly half its fibre (see recipe on page 238). You may also encounter chicory root as a caffeine-free coffee substitute.

JERUSALEM ARTICHOKES

Over 70% of the Jerusalem artichoke's fibre comes from inulin, making it one of the richest sources of this particular prebiotic. Some people call it 'fartichoke' because the high levels of non-digestible carbohydrate often lead to flatulence. If you aren't a regular vegetable eater or you have IBS, Jerusalem artichokes are probably best avoided. Otherwise, you might like to try our recipes for Jerusalem artichoke soup (see page 231) and Beef and Jerusalem artichoke casserole (see page 260).

WHOLEGRAINS

Wholegrains are also an important part of the traditional Mediterranean diet. Very low carbers may shun them, but wholegrains are full of the sort of fibre your good bacteria will love. The trouble with the grains we most commonly eat, such as wheat and rice, is that by the time they get to us most of the fibre and other nutrients have been stripped out. Switch from white to brown rice, and try adding a few other wholegrains to perk up your microbiome.

OATS

The most popular way to consume oats is in the form of porridge. Although I am a fan of porridge (we eat ours with added wheat bran and some toasted walnuts), I would urge you to avoid the highly processed instant stuff. You can cook proper porridge on the stove, or in the microwave, in a few minutes, or you might like to try our recipes on pages 225–6.

BARLEY

Barley is an ancient and very tasty grain, with a slightly nutty flavour. It is good in soups and stews. Barley scores well as a prebiotic because, like oats, it contains lots of beta-glucan. Beta-glucan is a soluble fibre that's been shown not just to boost your biome but to improve your cholesterol levels. It binds cholesterol in your gut, preventing it from being absorbed.

FLAXSEEDS

This is another healthy prebiotic, a seed with a slight, but not overwhelming, nutty flavour. You can scatter them on your porridge in the morning, or add them, toasted, to salads for a delicious crunch. They are rich in insoluble fibre, so as well as feeding your microbiome, they should help ensure regular bowel movements.

FRUIT

Apples and pears are high in microbiome-friendly fibre, particularly if you eat the skin. A medium-sized apple with its skin has 4 grams of fibre, while a medium-sized pear has 5 grams. I love stewed apples, with yoghurt, or diced and cooked in the oven with a scattering of cinnamon. We don't bother peeling them, even in a crumble.

Strawberries, blackberries and raspberries are also surprisingly high in fibre and low in sugar. They're an excellent source of vitamin C and contain decent amounts of folate (vitamin B9).

SEAWEED

Slippery, slimy, and with a very distinctive ocean flavour, seaweed is certainly an acquired taste. The seaweeds you are most likely to have encountered are nori, which is used to make sushi; dulse, which I was told tastes like bacon when fried – it doesn't; and kelp, which is used as a gluten-free alternative to noodles. Seaweeds are excellent prebiotics, packed with vitamins and minerals, as well as fibre, and probably the best source of omega-3 fatty acids. If only they didn't taste quite so strong...

COCOA

I am a hopeless chocaholic and will eat bars of it given a chance. Although milk chocolate, which is stuffed with fat and sugar, is clearly bad for us, cocoa itself is surprisingly healthy. Unsweetened cocoa powder contains more than 30% fibre and it is an excellent source of flavonoids and polyphenols, both good for your gut bacteria.

PREBIOTIC CAPSULES

I am normally very sceptical about the benefits of swallowing vitamin pills, fish oil capsules or supplements of any type. But a few years ago, I did agree, as part of a film I was making about sleep, to try out a product called Bimuno. This is a fibre supplement containing a prebiotic called galactooligosaccharide (GOS). There is good evidence that regular consumption will increase levels of the good bugs in your gut, such as *Bifidobacterium*. It is primarily taken to help with gut problems, but under the guidance of Professor Phil Burnet, a neuroscientist based at Oxford University who specialises in the effects of gut bacteria and prebiotics on brain function, I decided to see if it would have any impact on my sleep.

Phil provided me with a special sleep tracker which I wore for a week (to determine my baseline). Then I consumed the Bimuno powder for a couple of weeks (it comes in a sachet and you stir it into a cup of tea or milk). Then I stopped taking it.

At the end of my little self-experiment, I sent the tracker back to Phil and a few days later met up with him to discuss my results.

Despite my scepticism, consuming the powder did seem to have made a difference. I noticed that I had begun sleeping better a few days after starting taking it, and then reverted to my more normal restlessness a few days after stopping. And that is also what the tracker showed.

As Phil explained, 'If we look at the days before you took the supplement, 79% of your time in bed was spent sleeping and 21% of your time in bed was spent awake.' In other words, my sleep efficiency was a lousy 79%.

'But five days after taking the supplement', Phil went on, 'your sleep efficiency went up to 92%, which is an impressive turnaround. One thing that I was puzzled by was that on this night' – he pointed at my graph – 'your sleep efficiency suddenly went down; do you know what you were doing?'

'I went out and had a few drinks,' I admitted. 'I wondered at the time whether you'd notice.'

Is drinking a white powder the only way to get decent amounts of GOS? Phil suggested that I might get similar results from eating lentils, chickpeas, butter beans, lima beans and cashew nuts, but because the powder contains higher doses, obtaining it through food might take longer to have an effect.

When the sleep film went out in the UK, there was a big rush to buy Bimuno products. In fact, I still, occasionally, get stopped in the street by people who say they saw the programme and started taking Bimuno, and that it has transformed their sleep. Others, however, said it had made them windy, and it certainly can inflame the guts of people with IBS.

Probiotics

Just as important as feeding our microbiome with prebiotics is ensuring that we have the right balance of gut-friendly microbes in the first place. This is where probiotics come in. Probiotics are live bacteria or yeast that you parachute into your intestine, in the hope that they will take root and enrich your microbiome. There are lots of probiotic capsules and supplements out there, but as I've said before, I prefer topping up my 'good bacteria' through food.

YOGHURT

Yoghurt is a key part of the Mediterranean diet and it is also a good source of the probiotic *Lactobacillus*. I like full-fat, plain, Greek yoghurt. I add fruits to sweeten it, or scatter cinnamon, flaxseeds and nuts over it.

CHEESE

Like milk and yoghurt, I prefer my cheese full fat and unadulterated. Although I don't believe that eating cheese will give you nightmares, I would recommend you don't eat it close to bedtime. Not all cheese contains live bacteria, and processed cheese contains hardly any. You will find significant numbers of 'good' bacteria in Gouda, mozzarella, Cheddar and cottage cheese, as well as in blue cheese such as Roquefort.

FERMENTED FOODS

You can ferment almost anything, from vegetables to fish, but if you are not familiar with fermented foods, I would stick to some of the more standard ones, like sauerkraut or kimchi. They are particularly delicious when they are homemade. Clare describes how to do this in the *Clever Guts* books, and there are a couple of new recipes in the recipe section on page 223.

Although having a more diverse microbiome seems to help sleep, there is not a lot of research out there showing whether probiotics themselves have an impact. I've seen one study from Japan[78] which found that women eating fermented foods during pregnancy were more likely to have babies that sleep soundly during their first year of life (the baby gets its microbiome from mum), but unless you are used to them I would be cautious about including a lot of fermented foods when pregnant. Anecdotally, I've heard it helps some people but disrupts sleep in others.

PROBIOTIC CAPSULES

As with probiotic foods, there is not a lot of research on the impact of probiotics on sleep. I found one small study, published in March 2019 by neuroscientists based at the University of Verona, in Italy.[79] They asked 38 male and female students to consume a probiotic capsule containing a mixture of four different bacteria (*Lactobacillus fermentum*, *L. rhamnosus*, *L. plantarum* and *Bifidobacterium longum*) or a placebo, every day for six weeks. The students didn't know which they were getting.

The students filled in questionnaires that assessed their mood and how well they were sleeping at the beginning, middle and end of the experiment.

The scientists found that, unlike those swallowing placebo capsules, the students who were taking the probiotics saw modest improvements in both mood and sleep quality.

> **Caution for those with IBS, gut problems or reduced immunity**
>
> I mentioned earlier that for some people it takes time to boost a healthy microbiome, and if you are not used to eating fibre you may get some flatulence, bloating and possibly a bit of diarrhoea. This usually settles down – just build up your fibre intake slowly. However, those with IBS may need to proceed more cautiously or avoid adding fibre and fermented foods. If your immunity is suppressed, check with your doctor first.

Time-restricted eating

In the last chapter, I suggested that you might want to try this very popular form of intermittent fasting by having your evening meal a bit earlier and your breakfast a bit later. Practising TRE really can improve the quality of your shut-eye.

In a recent study run by scientists from the Salk Institute,[80] over-weight volunteers who restricted their eating to a 10-hour window (14:10) lost an average of 3.3kg over the course of 12 weeks. They also saw big reductions in waist size, blood sugar levels, blood pressure and 'bad cholesterol' levels. Last, and by no means least, most of them also enjoyed longer and less interrupted sleep.

Getting used to TRE can take time, but most people find that they soon adapt. I suggest you start by going 12 hours without eating (12:12) and then try to extend your overnight fast to 14 hours, i.e. 14:10.

Summary

Changing what you eat and when you eat can help you to sleep better:
- Try not to eat within three hours of bedtime.
- Experiment with extending your overnight fast to 12 and then to 14 hours.
- Cut back on sugar, sugary treats, drinks and desserts, particularly shop-bought ones. They lead to more fragmented sleep.
- Get more fibre into your diet by switching to brown rice, and by

eating more quinoa, bulgur, whole rye, wholegrain barley, wild rice, buckwheat, lentils and beans.

- Porridge oats are great for breakfast, as long as they are not the processed instant sort.

- Full-fat yoghurt is a good source of probiotics. Add blackberries, strawberries or blueberries for flavour. Or a sprinkling of nuts.

- Snack on nuts: they are a great source of protein and fibre, which should lead to more deep sleep. Try to avoid salted or sweetened nuts, which can be moreish.

- Eat oily fish such as salmon, tuna and mackerel, which are rich in omega-3 fatty acids, two to three times a week. An experiment conducted with American prisoners found that eating oily fish can improve sleep.

- The best fruits to give your biome a treat are berries, apples and pears.

- Have an alcoholic drink, if you must, but only with your evening meal. Try to average no more than a glass a day and try sticking to red wine, which studies have shown is better for you than white.

PART TWO:
The 4-Week Sleep Plan

7. The plan in practice

I've given you the latest science and identified some of the issues that prevent you from getting to sleep and staying asleep, along with advice on how to improve your sleep hygiene. I'm now going to pull all this information together into a four-week plan. Follow it, and you will soon be feeling far more cheerful, with more energy and greater mental clarity.

One of the first things you should be thinking about now is whether you want to try Sleep Restriction Therapy (SRT), the part of the plan that I introduced you to in Chapter 5.

SRT is extremely effective, but it is a challenge. Initially, during the day, you may feel sleepier and more irritable, so you do have to be very careful about driving or working machinery. Staying up late at night when you want to be asleep is also quite boring. The good news is that it doesn't last for long and it really does work.

Note: if you think you might have a significant health problem, or a sleep disorder such as sleep apnoea, consult your doctor before starting on a new programme such as this one. SRT should not be tried by pregnant women or young children.

Before you start

As the American president Abraham Lincoln once said: 'Give me six hours to chop down a tree and I will spend the first four sharpening the axe.' The following is a list of things I recommend you do before you start the plan.

KEEP A SLEEP DIARY

Below is a sample page from a sleep diary. You can download and print a similar one from my website, www.fast-asleep.com/sleep-diary/. I want you to fill in your sleep diary for a week before you start the programme and then every week during the course.

The point of keeping a sleep diary is to assess how well you are sleeping and to help you calculate your sleep efficiency, i.e. the amount of time you spend in bed actually asleep. Just to remind you, if you are in bed for eight hours but asleep for six hours, then you have an efficiency rating of $6/8 = 0.75$ or 75%, which is poor.

By the end of the four weeks, you should be aiming to get it up to 85%; 100% is unrealistic because everyone needs a bit of time to drift off. If you are falling asleep immediately when your head hits the pillow, I would be worried that you are too sleep deprived.

If you don't get as high as 85%, don't worry. An efficiency rating of 80% is perfectly acceptable, particularly for older people.

How to estimate how long you have slept: if you have a sleep tracker it will do this for you. I have found that mine takes a lot of the stress out of recording my sleep patterns. It will also track your heart rate, making it more accurate than a device that simply records your movements. If you don't have a tracker, you simply take the time you went to bed, the time you woke, and take away roughly how long you were awake during the night. In other words, if you went to bed at 11pm, got up at 7am and were awake for two hours during the night, that means you were asleep for eight hours minus two hours = six hours.

How to calculate your sleep efficiency: in brief, take the amount of time you were asleep, turn it into minutes and divide by the time you were in bed (again in minutes). In this case it would be 360/480 = 75%. Remember, you are aiming for 85%.

PURCHASE ANY SLEEP AIDS

If you want to try some of the supplements I've written about, order them online now because they will take a while to arrive. If you live in the UK, Bimuno will be delivered in a few days, but melatonin ordered from the US will take at least a week.

You can buy a light box from a shop or online, but make sure you choose one that provides 10,000 lux and has some decent ratings.

SLEEP DIARY

(to be filled in once you are fully awake in the morning)

Date	Mon	Tue	Wed	Thu	Fri	Sat	Sun
Before bed							
What time was your last food or drink?							
When was your last coffee or tea?							
How many alcoholic drinks did you have?							
During the night							
When did you go to bed?							
Did you find it hard to fall asleep?							
Did you wake in the night?							
If so, how often?							
And for how long?							
What time did you get up?							
Estimate how long you slept							

Date	Mon	Tue	Wed	Thu	Fri	Sat	Sun
Calculate your sleep efficiency							
Rate your sleep, 1-5							
How tired are you, 1-5?							
Thinking about yesterday							
Did you fall asleep unintentionally?							
How many coffees did you have?							
Did you have an afternoon slump?							
Were you irritable?							
Did you exercise?							
Food and drink							
Are you eating more fibre-rich foods?							
Are you eating/ drinking more fermented foods?							

MEASURE YOUR WEIGHT, WAIST AND BLOOD SUGAR LEVELS

I think it is very motivating to be able to measure the effect that improved sleep is having on your health, as well as your energy levels. I would expect your food cravings to reduce as you begin to sleep better, and for your waist and neck to shrink. So why not whip out a tape measure and measure both right now?

You measure your waist by wrapping the tape around your belly button, not your hips. Why is waist size important? Because it is an indirect measure of your visceral, internal fat and one of the best predictors we have of future health. Ideally, it should be less than half your height (so if you are 6 feet or 182cm tall your waist should be less than 36 inches, or 91cm).

Having too much fat around the neck is bad because it can affect breathing and lead to snoring and sleep apnoea. If you are a man, it should measure less than 17 inches (43cm), for a woman less than 16 inches (41cm). Losing an inch or more around your neck could make a huge difference to your sleep and the quality of your life.

I would also recommend you measure your blood sugar levels, as blood sugar control is badly affected by poor sleep. Sleep deprivation not only increases the stress hormone cortisol (which messes up your blood sugar levels) but also acts on hunger hormones like leptin and ghrelin, which will then cause you to overeat. Around one in three adults in the UK have prediabetes (raised blood sugar levels, not yet in the diabetic range) and most don't know they have it. Chronic insomnia raises your risk of prediabetes and type 2 diabetes, particularly if you are under 40.

The only way to tell if your blood sugars are abnormal is to measure them. You can ask your GP to test you, or you can do it yourself with a digital blood sugar monitoring kit, which you can buy quite cheaply at a chemist or online.

If they are currently raised, I would expect to see both your blood sugars and your blood pressure improve as you begin to sleep better.

If I'm overweight, should I prioritise improving sleep or losing weight?

If you are significantly overweight, you might be wondering whether to sort out your weight or your sleep first. You can do both at the same time. Losing weight will help you sleep better, while sleeping better will make losing inches around your waist and neck that much easier. Tackling both at the same time is certainly doable, though a challenge. The good news is that the recipes in this book, based on a low-carb Mediterranean diet, discussed in Chapter 6, are not only great for helping your sleep but will also help keep you fuller for longer, which in turn will help you shed fat and keep it off.

Many people have told me that time-restricted eating (TRE), see page 166, which I write about extensively in my most recent book, *The Fast 800*, has helped them lose weight and improved their sleep. So do give it a go.

GET COOKING AND FERMENTING!

Feeding up your microbiome by eating more fibre-rich and fermented foods is an important part of this plan, so take a look at our recipes and see which ones you fancy trying over the coming weeks. If your diet isn't currently fibre-rich, introduce these foods gradually as otherwise you will start producing a lot of gas!

You can buy fermented foods in the shops, but making your own sauerkraut is relatively easy and very rewarding. Just bear in mind that it will take time to mature.

SORT OUT YOUR BEDROOM

Ensure that your bedroom is a place where you sleep and have sex, nothing more. So:

- If you have a TV in your bedroom, take it out;
- Replace any bright lights with bulbs that are softer and more diffuse;
- If you like the idea of music or white noise to fall asleep to, now is the time to get everything set up.

How's your mattress?

As a rule of thumb, you should replace your mattress every seven to ten years, but the life expectancy of a mattress varies considerably, depending on how good it was in the first place and how much of a pounding it has had. The main thing to watch out for is sagging. Take the sheets off and have a good look to see whether there is an obvious dip. If there is, a mattress topper will provide extra cushion and support and will be much cheaper than a new mattress.

What sort of pillow is best?

In theory, you should replace your pillow every couple of years. To test if it is time for a new one, try folding it in half and see if it springs open. If it doesn't, it probably won't be providing a lot of support for your head and neck.

If you do decide to replace it, what sort of pillow should you buy? According to the National Sleep Foundation (NSF) that depends on how you sleep.

People who sleep on their back will benefit from thinner pillows 'which help to limit stress on the neck'. Stomach sleepers need a really thin pillow, or no pillow at all, to keep the spine straight and minimise stress on the lower back. For side sleepers (the most popular position), a standard pillow will do, though they might consider 'placing a pillow between their knees or thighs to help maintain spinal alignment as they sleep'.

Keep it dark

Finally, do make sure that your room is cool, dark and quiet. If you have a clock, put it away, out of sight. Your mobile should, ideally, be switched off or placed face down on a table that is out of reach of your bed. You might want to invest in decent curtains or blackout blinds, particularly if you are a shift worker, though a sleep mask will be a good deal cheaper.

With all that sorted, it's time to take the plunge and get started. As I have said, the 4-Week Sleep Plan will be particularly helpful if you suffer from insomnia, but it will also benefit those of you who experience occasional disrupted sleep.

If you don't fancy sleep restriction, or you give it a go and find it too hard, do try the other key aspects of the plan – practising good sleep hygiene, changing the way you eat to create a sleepy biome and doing your best to combat stress and anxiety to remain worry-free during the night.

Week one

Priorities for the week

Your main priorities for the first week are, firstly, to make sure you fill in your sleep diary every day. I find the best time to do this is first thing in the morning and, despite some reservations about sleep trackers, I do think they can be extremely useful when you are trying to work out when you fell asleep and how many hours you slept the previous night.

Your sleep diary is an essential tool if you want to understand why you are struggling to sleep and what you can do about it.

Your next priority is to choose a wake-up time and stick to it, at weekends as well as during the week. Setting a fixed wake-up time is a vital way of anchoring your sleep and letting your brain and body know who is in charge. You will be strongly tempted to have lie-ins, but try to resist. I am only asking you to commit to trying this for four weeks, and I think that is a small price to pay if you want to wake up feeling rested in the future, rather than shattered.

Your third priority is to make sure that your bedroom is sorted and there are no distracting electronics around. I don't expect you to keep your mobile phone in another room (though some people do) but do at least try to keep it out of reach. I keep mine on a chest of drawers well out of the way. Since I also use my mobile as an alarm clock, that means I have to get out of bed to turn it off.

Avoid keeping your phone by your bed as you will be tempted to pick it up and start scrolling. According to Google Trends the most popular time of day for people to search for the word 'Insomnia' is at 3am, which is deeply ironic as they are presumably searching for solutions to their insomnia on their smart phones.

I would hope that by now you will have read through and tried out a few of the recipes in the back of the book. Changing your diet will have a big effect on the quality of your sleep, as will practising time-restricted eating (where you stop eating 3 hours before you go to bed). So do give it a go.

I repeat again: for those of you who feel that sleep restriction therapy is something you would like to try, then keeping a sleep diary, noting when you go to bed, when you get up and how many hours you spent awake is an absolute must. Only when you have recorded a full week of how you are currently sleeping can you decide how much you are going to restrict and measure your progress.

THE 4-WEEK SLEEP PLAN – WEEK ONE

I have introduced you to all the basic principles you need to improve your sleep. Which you use and how you use them is, of course, entirely up to you. I have, nonetheless, put together a four-week plan to remind you about some of the things I have already discussed, with suggestions as to how and when to put them into practice. Use them as a guide, but do put your own particular spin on them and try as many as you like each day.

MONDAY

The previous night you will have set your alarm to wake you up at the perfect time in the morning, one that will give you enough time to get up and get ready for the day ahead, but not so early that you can't stick with it long term. This is the number one rule of every sleep expert I have spoken to, which is why I am repeating it yet again.

Sorting out your insomnia and improving your sleep depends on keeping your wake-up time the same, whether it is during the week or at the weekend. So, when the alarm rings, do get out of bed!

The next thing I want you to do is fill in your sleep diary. This, as I've stressed earlier, is essential if you are to get a real understanding of how much of your time you spend in bed asleep, rather than just lying there tossing and turning.

When you do get up, how about going for a brisk early morning walk before breakfast? This way you not only get the advantages of a bit of morning exercise, but exposure to bright light that will help reset your body clock for the day ahead.

Going for a brisk walk (or some other form of workout) will also delay when you have breakfast, and when you drink coffee.

Remember, it is best not to drink coffee within an hour of waking, and best to have it with your breakfast.

If you are thinking of trying time-restricted eating (TRE – see page 166), then why not start today by doing 12:12? That means eating within a 12-hour time window, for example between 8am and 8pm. Your goal should be to finish your evening meal at least three hours before you go to bed and avoid snacking before going to sleep.

TUESDAY

If you haven't already done so, now is a good time to start following a more Mediterranean diet (which means lots of olive oil, nuts, oily fish, fruit, vegetables and wholegrains), as studies show a high M score (ticking as many Mediterranean diet boxes as possible) leads to longer and better sleep. A good place to start might be with Rosy overnight oats (page 226), which combines berries, oats, almonds, apricots and Greek yoghurt. The great thing is you can prepare this the night before.

Another good thing about oats is that they contain a particular type of fibre which is not only good for sleep but has also been shown to lower cholesterol in just 4 weeks.

WEDNESDAY

How about starting a 'to-do' journal (see page 123)? The idea is that keeping a 'to-do' journal should stop you worrying at 3am, about things you need to do the following morning. Another technique that some experts swear by is a '30-minute worry'. A couple of hours before bed you set aside 30 minutes or so to think about all the things that are worrying you and focus on those. It might seem a bit self-indulgent, but better that you worry in the early evening than in the middle of the night.

THURSDAY

Today I would like you to practise some of the simple breathing exercises which I wrote about earlier (see page 130). I have personally found them to be a real game changer, a wonderful way to calm myself down when I'm stressed, and a great way to help ease me back to sleep when I wake up in the middle of the night. The simplest approach is 4-2-4 (inhale for a count of four, hold for two, then exhale for four), but you may prefer one of the other variants. Slowing down your breathing sounds ridiculously simple but it is incredibly effective. That said, you must practise during the day when you are not stressed, otherwise you may find it hard to do it at night.

FRIDAY

I recommend you start the day with some resistance exercises, like press-ups and squats, and to get outside for a blast of sunlight in the morning – even if it's a cloudy day (see page 136). If you have decided to try a SAD light, this might be a good day to start using it. Remember, no caffeine for the first hour of the day, and no caffeine after 12pm. If you are trying to stick to TRE (time-restricted eating) then that also means no alcohol within 3 hours of going to bed.

SATURDAY

Don't hit the snooze button on your alarm! It might be the weekend but I'm afraid a luxurious lie-in is out of the question. Weekend lie-ins will mess up your circadian rhythms which are so important to drive the urge to sleep.

Why not take advantage of the extra time (particularly if everyone else in the house is still sleeping) to get busy in the kitchen making a batch of home-made Purple pickled onions? Clare's recipe (page 290) is really easy to make and packed with far more healthy bugs than most supermarket alternatives. It only takes a few minutes, and it will be thoroughly fermented and bursting with sleep-inducing beneficial bacteria within five to ten days.

SUNDAY

That is the first week almost done. So, how did it go? Did you manage to fill in your sleep diary? If so, use it to calculate your sleep efficiency. If you are starting sleep restriction therapy next week, then work out when you are going to go to bed, what you are planning to do while everyone else in the house is asleep, and make sure that it fits in with your schedule over the next few weeks. You don't want to start sleep restriction if you are going to be doing a lot of driving or if you have work commitments which require you to be totally on the ball. Sleep restriction is tough, at least initially, and you will feel tired.

Sunday is also a good day to plan and even prepare healthy meals for the following week. Clare has included a selection of healthy lunch recipes at the back of this book which will expand your packed lunch horizons (and significantly boost your nutrient intake), like Prawns and red cabbage slaw on sourdough (page 250) or Smoked mackerel, beetroot and tahini pitta (page 251).

By the end of the first week, it is possible that simply by practising the principles of sleep hygiene you will already be sleeping better. I recently met a woman called Jayne who said she hadn't had a decent night's sleep since she gave birth to her first child, thirty years ago. She had seen an article I'd written about sleep, decided to give up late-night snacking and alcohol, had put aside 15 minutes at 9pm to write down her worries and concerns, and also to reflect on good things that had happened to her that day. She said that just doing these simple things had been enough to transform her sleep.

One week down, three to go! How many these have you introduced this week?	
Sleep diary	
Morning walk	
Time-restricted eating	
Mediterranean-inspired meals	
'To-do' journal	
Breathing exercises	
Resistance training	
Early weekend wake up	

SLEEP RESTRICTION THERAPY – HOW TO DO IT

Now that you have filled in a full week of your sleep diary, it's time to try Sleep Restriction Therapy, if you have discovered in week one that you are lying in bed awake for long periods of the night. First of all, you need to plan how many hours you are going to spend in bed for the next week – i.e. by how much you are going to restrict your sleep window.

Let's assume you currently go to bed at 11pm and get out of bed at 7am. But though you lie in bed for eight hours, your tracker shows that you only sleep, on average, for six hours, giving you a sleep efficiency of 75%, which, you'll recall, is low.

Having established that you sleep for six hours, starting with week 2 you are going to spend just six hours in bed each night. You will get up at the same time every morning, i.e. at 7am. But instead of going to bed at 11pm, you are going to go to bed at 1am. (Similarly, if you have found that you are only asleep for five and a half hours, then for the next week you are going to spend just five and a half hours in bed; and so you will go to bed at 1.30am.)

The four main rules, if you decide to try SRT, are:

1. Do not cut your time in bed to below five hours.
2. Stick to it rigorously.
3. Do not lie down, nap or snooze during the day and get your family to wake you if you do.
4. Do not drive or use machinery if you experience serious daytime sleepiness.

How long do I do it for?

SRT may radically improve your sleep in a couple of weeks, or it may take up to 8 weeks to be fully effective. As your sleep efficiency improves you increase the amount of time you spend in bed until you feel you are getting sufficient sleep.

If, as in the example above, you have cut the time you spend in bed to six hours then you should find, after a few days, that although you are spending less time in bed, you are spending more of that time sleeping. So you are now in bed for six hours, but perhaps sleeping for five hours. In which case your sleep efficiency is now 5/6 = 83%. Once it has got to 85% or better, for several nights in a row, you can move your bedtime to 20 minutes earlier.

Why 20 minutes? Why not 30 minutes? Or 40 minutes? There are different views, with some experts saying the increments should be in blocks of 15 minutes, and others suggesting blocks of 30 minutes work best; 20 minutes is a compromise.

Getting to 85% will probably take a week. If it doesn't start to improve after a week, you may need to cut your time in bed even further. In this example, you would go down to five hours and 40 minutes, going to bed at 1.20am. If that doesn't do it, you could reduce it again, but I would be inclined to consult a doctor because it could mean you have a more complex problem.

Remember, never go below five hours in bed. Assuming, like most people, that you have reached your 85% target after the first week of the course, then for the second week you will be going to bed for six hours and 20 minutes. Your sleep efficiency may initially drop below 85% for a while. If it does, keep going with this new regime until it is once more reliably back above 85%. This may take another week. When it is above 85%, add another 20 minutes to your sleep schedule. And so on, until you feel that you are getting not only enough sleep, but enough good-quality sleep.

You will know this is happening because you will wake up feeling more refreshed, you will have less daytime sleepiness and you will be able to pass the Spoon Test (page 89).

Some people will find three weeks of SRT is enough, but it can take up to eight weeks if you have serious long-term insomnia.

SRT is tough, particularly for the first week. You will probably feel more tired during the day than you do at the moment. You will feel moody, and you may struggle to be sociable. You will almost certainly get the munchies.

You must tell your friends, family and colleagues at work, what you are doing, and why you are doing it, so they know why you are more sleepy, forgetful and bad-tempered than normal. Try not to compensate by increasing your caffeine intake. And don't nap! This would be a bad time to go to the cinema, the theatre, or anywhere warm and dark where you might nod off. You may find it easier to adhere to the course with professional support from a practitioner who is trained in delivering CBTi (Cognitive Behavioural Therapy for insomnia). Find out more at https://www.babcp.com

What should I do between 11pm and 1am?
You might think that with all that extra time you have during the night, you will be able do lots of useful or creative activities. But when I tried SRT I didn't do anything particularly productive. I read a lot of books, and I watched a lot of TV. Although TV in the bedroom isn't a great

idea, it is fine to watch it in the living room. But don't fall asleep and do make sure you go to bed when you are supposed to.

What is the evidence that it works?

Sleep restriction is not new. It was first tested as a way of treating insomnia in the 1980s by an American psychologist called Arthur Spielman. In a now classic study, published in 1987,[81] he got 35 middle-aged patients who had been chronic insomniacs for more than 15 years and asked them to sleep restrict for up to eight weeks.

Before they started, the insomniacs were spending an average of eight hours in bed but, despite taking sleeping pills, they were only sleeping for 5 hours and 20 minutes. In other words, they were tossing and turning for an average of 2 hours and 40 minutes every night. Their sleep efficiency was a miserable 67%.

Spielman didn't ask them to do anything else apart from cutting down to an average of 5 hours and 40 minutes in bed each night, slowly increasing that amount as the weeks went by.

The results were amazing (remember these were chronic insomniacs, most of whom had been taking sleeping pills for over 15 years).

Within a week they reported improved sleep. Over the course of the study their sleep efficiency improved from 67% to 87%. By the end of eight weeks they were spending 90 minutes less time in bed each night, but sleeping for longer than before. What I find particularly impressive is that the amount of time they spent awake, in bed, fretting, was down by almost two hours! Even better, unlike drugs, doing sleep restriction had long lasting results with no side effects. In a follow-up study carried out nine months later almost all of them had managed to keep their insomnia at bay.

Spielman's experiment has been repeated many times and a recent meta-analysis[82] showed very clearly that this technique works: cutting down time spent in bed really does reset the brain. People sleep more deeply, wake up less often and feel much better during the day.

What are the benefits?

Firstly, your sleep improves really fast. People who've followed my advice and tried SRT say they're astonished how quickly they began to sleep much more deeply, which in turn improved their mood. They no longer worried about 'not going to sleep' when they went to bed. Instead, they yearned for bed, fell asleep rapidly and were much less likely to wake up during the night.

Interestingly, restricting sleep has also been shown to be a swift and effective way of treating depression. A recent review of 66 studies[83] looking into the impact of sleep restriction on different forms of depression found that around half of patients with depression (particularly those who were bipolar) responded well to it, though many found it hard to maintain. Researchers are currently looking at how to combine it with bright light therapy.

Week two

Your priorities this week are to keep filling in your sleep diary and to continue getting out of bed at the same time in the morning, however sleepy you feel. In addition, here are a few questions to ask yourself at the start of week two.

SRT

If you have decided to give the sleep restriction regime a go, then are you properly prepared? Go back to page 187 to refresh your memory on how to do it. The week ahead will be challenging, but if it helps you crack your insomnia then it will be worth it.

CAFFEINE AND ALCOHOL

Did you try cutting back on these two sleep disrupters, and did it help? Depending on how much you were drinking, I would expect an alcohol-free week to have made a difference. If you can manage another week, I would stick to it. After all, this is a four-week plan and most people can manage a month without booze.

As for caffeine, hopefully you have found that you don't actually need it as much as you thought you did. Lots of people tell me that giving up one cup of coffee a day is no big deal and that, in the afternoon, a cup of tea, which is lighter on caffeine, fulfils much of the emotional need to give yourself a break.

TIME-RESTRICTED EATING

Did you give this a go, and did it help? Getting used to TRE can take time, but most people find that they soon adapt. If you have found it relatively easy to do 12:12, you may want to extend your overnight fast from 12 to 14 hours, i.e. 14:10. If, however, you have found it a struggle or it has made your sleep worse, it is perfectly OK to put this aside for now and try again in a few weeks' time. It is also OK to break the rules on a couple of occasions a week but try to maintain TRE five days a week.

Week two plan

MONDAY

Check in with your sleep efficiency – has it improved at all? I wouldn't expect miracles, but if you have been going out for those early morning walks and practising good sleep hygiene, I would expect some improvements. And if you have been doing the deep breathing exercises, then I hope you are finding them useful, particularly in the middle of the night. If you're still drinking a lot of caffeine, now is the time to start gradually weaning yourself off it. Cut down to 2–3 cups of coffee, maximum, and try drinking more herbal teas during the afternoons.

TUESDAY

As your sleep improves you should find your attitude towards bed improving too. When you spend hours and hours each night lying awake, tossing and turning, worrying about insomnia and anxious about how tired you're going to feel the next day, it can be easy to dread being in bed. But your bedroom should be a cosy haven that you love. So give your bedroom a good tidy, re-arrange the furniture if you think it might help, and consider investing in a face mask, or even a new pillow (in theory you should replace a pillow every two years).

WEDNESDAY

If your sleep has been fractured for some time you may have become reliant on sugary snacks to keep your energy levels up during the day, but highly processed foods and fizzy drinks will set you on a blood sugar rollercoaster that continues through the day and night, ultimately trapping you in a vicious cycle of sleeplessness. Take this opportunity to try to cut down on sugar and simple carbohydrates (shop-bought cakes and biscuits) but don't worry, treats aren't completely off the table if you bake a batch of Clare's delicious Zucchini, orange and apricot cakes (see page 286) – they are remarkably sweet (considering they don't contain any added sugar!) and packed with healthy fibre your sleep-friendly gut microbiome loves.

THURSDAY

If you are doing SRT, then resist the temptation to close your eyes, no matter how tired you feel during the day – for this plan to be really effective in the shortest possible time, you need to build up your sleep drive so you are ready to fall asleep the minute your head hits the pillow; to drift off easily when you wake up in the middle of the night; and to sleep solidly from then until your alarm goes off in the morning. So, be alert and don't let yourself drop off in the car or in front of the TV in the evening. If you are exhausted and you absolutely must nap, keep it short (no longer than 20 minutes) and no later than 3pm.

FRIDAY

If you want to celebrate approaching the end of week two, why not experiment with some of the wide range of alcohol-free drinks which are now available? Remember, drinking alcohol makes you more likely to make poor (and potentially sleep-sabotaging) food choices, and although you might think a few drinks will help you drop off, booze is only going to make you more likely to snore and it can lead to fragmented sleep later on. So, at least for now, say no to early evening cocktails and nightcaps before bed. The longer you can stay off alcohol, the more effective this sleep plan will be.

SATURDAY

Well done for making it through the week! Take a bit of time today to pat yourself on the back for the work you've put in to improving your sleep. The second week is often the toughest time, and things can only get better from here. Why not start your day with a nice indulgent breakfast, such as Scrambled eggs with kimchi (page 227) or Sweet potato savoury muffins with feta (page 228).

SUNDAY

Now that you are almost at the end of the first two weeks on this sleep plan, your sleep quality should be improving, and your energy levels should be creeping back up. This means, if you haven't already done so, it's time to incorporate more exercise into your routine – not just because exercise is very good for almost every aspect of your mental and physical health, but because it will improve your sleep as well.

EXERCISE

Becoming more active provides a huge range of health benefits, including improvements in mood and reductions in the risk of heart disease, cancer and stroke. I don't like doing exercise for its own sake, and I hate the gym, so I have found ways to build it into my life. I've included some simple resistance, aerobic and HIIT (High Intensity Interval Training) exercises to help you get going in weeks 2 and 3 of the plan.

Does it matter when I exercise?

It is best to exercise first thing, ideally in the early-morning light and ideally in the fasted state (i.e. before breakfast). We're told that we shouldn't exercise in the evening because it interferes with sleep, but there seems to be very little evidence for that. The important thing is you do it, so don't worry too much about whether the time is right.

Will it help me fall asleep, straight off?

Probably not. Doing more exercise and being more active will undoubtedly help you sleep better. But not immediately. In a small study,

70 researchers from Chicago asked 11 sedentary middle-aged women with insomnia to follow an exercise regime for 16 weeks.

To start with, they met a sleep expert, who gave them advice on sleep hygiene (going to bed and getting up at the same time every day, etc.).

They were also introduced to a personal trainer, who spent the next four months guiding them through an exercise regime. Four times a week, they had to do a 40-minute session in the gym, on a treadmill or an exercise bike, pushing themselves hard enough to get their heart rates up to around 120 beats per minute. So what happened?

At the beginning of the experiment, the women were in bed for an average of seven hours and 30 minutes, but only getting five hours and 54 minutes of actual sleep. By the end of the four months, they were getting 46 minutes more sleep per night.

The researchers found no direct link between the days on which the women had exercised and how they had slept that particular night. Instead, it was the other way around: after a bad night's sleep the women found it much harder to get motivated to exercise and they got exhausted much faster. Sticking to their exercise regime, when they were tired, became a struggle.

The moral is that you have to treat exercise as a way of life. The relationship between sleep and exercise is more of a virtuous circle than a quick fix. The other issue to be aware of is that when you don't want to exercise, you will find every excuse to avoid it. The lure of the TV and the sofa will be irresistible.

You have to find ways to do it, even if you are not in the mood. Whatever you do, don't rely on willpower! Willpower is grossly over-rated. Find something you actually like doing (Zumba? Swimming? Five-a-side football?) or make it something that is hard to avoid – park your car further away from your house, for example, so you are less tempted to jump into it for short journeys, or make a regular arrange-ment to run or train with a friend.

RESISTANCE EXERCISES

After the age of 30, most people start to lose muscle; if you are phys-ically inactive, it can be as much as 5% of your muscle mass for each decade that passes. Having more muscle means you look toned, plus it enables you to burn more calories and helps deep sleep. What's not to love? The best way to preserve your muscles is to do weight training or resistance exercises. I have a workout, which I call Fast Strength, and I try to do this most mornings. It works a range of muscles and takes only a few minutes. It is a combination of six exercises that work the top half (push-ups and triceps dips), the legs (squats and lunges) and the abs (crunches and the plank). You should aim to do 30 seconds of each, with 10 seconds rest in between. Repeat if you feel able.

Push-ups: lie face down with the palms of your hands under your shoulders and the balls of your feet touching the ground. Keep your body straight. Lower your body till your elbows form a right angle with the floor and then push up. If you find this too hard, do it with your knees on the ground.

Squats: stand with your feet apart. Bend from the hips, keeping the weight in your heels. Make sure your back is straight. Keep bending until your legs are at right angles to the floor – imagine you are preparing to sit in a chair. Push back up without bending your back. Squats work the biggest muscles in your body. You can make this harder by holding weights as you squat.

Crunches: lie on your back with your knees bent, your feet flat on the floor and your hands by the sides of your head. Curl up your upper body without lifting your lower back off the floor. Make sure your chin is tucked in towards your chest. When your shoulders and upper back are lifted off the floor, curl back down.

Plank: lie face down on the floor and then raise yourself on to your forearms and toes so that your body forms a straight line from head to toe. Make sure your midsection doesn't rise or drop. Squeeze your buttocks and hold the position for as long as possible. Remember, it should never cause pain in the lower back.

Lunges: stand with your back straight and your feet shoulder-width apart. Step forward with one leg, bending both knees to right angles and keeping your upper body straight. Pull back to the starting position and repeat, putting the other leg forward.

Triceps dips: stand with your back to a bench or chair. Place your palms on the seat behind you, bending your knees to right angles, hips straight. Bend your elbows to right angles to lower your body so that your bottom descends halfway to the floor. Push yourself back up using only your arms.

Recipe suggestions for week 2

- Nutty berry crunch (page 287)
- Roasted vegetables with thyme (page 278)
- Dr Tim's hot-smoked salmon salad (page 239)

Week three

Your priority, as for the previous weeks, is to make sure you are filling in your sleep diary and getting up at the same time every morning. Your sleep efficiency really should be steadily improving now. If it isn't, ask yourself what the barriers are. Have you been trying out the recipes? Practising the breathing exercises? Getting out of bed if you don't feel sleepy and only going back to bed when you do?

If you're doing Sleep Restriction Therapy and are now achieving an 85% sleep efficiency, it's time to reward yourself with an extra 20 minutes in bed. But don't be disappointed if you are not quite there. It can take up to eight weeks to transform your sleep, though most people see significant improvements in four.

Whatever stage you're at, it's also a good idea to stop talking about sleep. If someone asks how the programme is going, say 'great, thanks' (even if you're having a tricky day). By channelling positive thoughts, you can dial down some of the stress and negativity you might have associated with sleep, slow the negative spirals, and work towards thinking of yourself as 'sometimes' having trouble sleeping, rather than slipping into the self-fulfilling prophecy that can come with labelling yourself an 'insomniac'.

MONDAY

Have you been practising stimulus control? This basically means retraining your body to associate bed with sleep and sex and nothing else (see page 130). So if you don't feel sleepy, don't go to bed until you do. And if you wake up in the middle of the night and can't get back to sleep, get out of bed and find something dull to do until you feel like you are tired enough to fall straight asleep when you climb back into bed.

TUESDAY

I want you to really boost your M score by adding legumes (peas, beans, lentils) and wholegrains to your meals – do it gradually so your gut has a chance to adapt. Your microbiome LOVES pulses and 'good' gut bacteria manufacture the feel-good hormone, serotonin, which plays a role in regulating appetite, digestion and significantly – sleep. So experiment with using a white bean mash to top Shepherd's pie rather than potato (page 269) or adding lentils to your Bolognese sauce (see turkey and lentil bolognese, page 272).

WEDNESDAY

As well as writing in a 'worry journal' each day to help you offload the anxiety that can start to build before bed, why not also try counting your blessings? There is solid science behind the claim that getting into the habit of being regularly grateful not only makes you feel happier, but can also improve your sleep. The idea behind 'Three Good Things' is that you jot down in a notebook three things that happened that day which you are thankful for. Perhaps someone showed you kindness, or you saw a beautiful sunset or you had a good laugh with a friend. Just write it down and reflect on it. The aim of regular gratitude practice is to develop a 'grateful mindset' which can have powerfully positive effects on your mood. And your sleep.

THURSDAY

As well as doing slow deep breathing, one of the best ways to lull yourself back to sleep if you do find yourself awake in the middle of the night, is a mindfulness technique called Progressive Muscle Relaxation (see page 207). It's very easy, and increasingly powerful the more you do it. So do give it a go. But be aware, it does require practice, so best to learn how to do it during the day, rather than flipping desperately through this book in the middle of the night.

FRIDAY

How are you doing with your exercise regime? I strongly recommend a morning walk, to expose yourself to bright light, but if you can't get outside then doing some resistance exercises first thing, like press-ups and squats, is just as good. They are not only brilliant for your muscles and brain, but also good for your spine. The secret to acquiring a new habit that sticks is consistency, but also 'hooking' it to something you are already doing. You have to get out of bed every morning, so why not do some press-ups and squats when you do? Start gently and build up. According to a study presented at the American Heart Association's Health Conference in March 2022, people who started doing more resistance exercises increased the amount of good quality sleep they got by an average of 40 minutes.

SATURDAY

You're coming to the end of week three – that's amazing! Tonight it's time to treat yourself to a luxuriously pampering warm bath with a few drops of lavender essential oil (vanilla, rose and bergamot oils can also be effective) and play some relaxing music. A bath time ritual like this can help prime your body and brain for sleep. For the best results, time your bath for an hour before bedtime and soak yourself for at least 10 minutes. This means your body will be cooling down nicely as you get into bed.

SUNDAY

Make sure you're still getting up with your alarm each morning – even though it's the weekend. It might seem ridiculously early but think of all you can achieve in this extra time! You can start by running through the series of simple exercises I put my body through each morning (see page 199) because resistance exercises are a great way of improving the quality of your sleep further.

Then why not mark the end of week three by baking a cake? Clare's Dorset apple cake (page 284) is deliciously tangy and sweetened with gut-friendly dates instead of sugar.

Techniques to slow down your racing mind

Anyone who has wrestled with their sleep will be familiar with the feeling that your brain has gone into overdrive just as you want it to switch off. An overactive brain is often the product of physical and psychological forces. Changing what you eat and when you eat should improve your microbiome and help reduce feelings of anxiety. But there are lots of other things you can do that will help.

As I mentioned earlier, one of the main things that keeps people awake at night is worrying about staying awake and the terrible consequences of not getting to sleep. Thoughts like: 'I won't get to sleep and if I don't then I will feel really tired at work tomorrow and get the sack.'

It's important to realise that these thoughts are not real. They are not statements of fact. They can be challenged. You might want to give your negative thoughts a name, like 'Donald'. So when you have them you can say: 'That is just Donald sounding off again.'

Challenging yourself sounds crazy, but it works. The other key point to remember is that the negative thoughts you have at night are even less rooted in reality than the negative thoughts you have during the day. The filters are down, and you are more vulnerable to your inner demons.

You should also be aware that being sleep deprived will make you more prone to repetitive Automatic Negative Thoughts (ANTs), along the lines of 'I'm a failure, no one loves me', etc. Once your sleep improves, you will find that whenever you have ANTs they will be easier to stamp out.

Another way of approaching your catastrophic or negative thoughts is by imagining how a sympathetic friend would respond if you were to share them. What would they say? How would they help to ground you? As well as learning how to challenge these thoughts (which may well involve seeing a therapist), you can break the cycle by getting up and distracting yourself (reading a book, listening to music) or you can learn how to acknowledge them but then let them go by practising mindfulness (see page 208).

Another technique that some people find helpful is something called 'Paradoxical intention', where you deliberately try to stay awake when you are desperate to go to sleep. So, rather than stressing yourself by thinking, 'I must go to sleep now', you say to yourself, 'I am enjoying being awake. I really am. Let's see how long I can stay awake for.' It takes the pressure off and by doing so it can, paradoxically, lead to sleep.

Breathing and progressive muscle relaxation

Although I like the idea of paradoxical intention, I personally find doing breathing and progressive muscle relaxation exercises more effective when I am struggling to sleep. As well as the 4-2-4 technique I described on page 131, you could try alternate-nostril breathing. This is the basis of a well-known yogic exercise, known as nadi shodhana pranayama, meaning 'subtle energy clearing breathing technique'.

Start by breathing out through your mouth and then use your right thumb to close your right nostril.

Breathe in deeply through your left nostril to a count of four. Really fill your belly. Now switch sides. Block your left nostril with your left thumb and breathe out fully to a count of four. Repeat 10 times.

If you feel at all dizzy, which I did the first time I attempted this, you are trying too hard. Don't push yourself. This is supposed to be relaxing.

Progressive muscle relaxation is another exercise that anyone can do, but it would be a good idea to practise doing it a few times during the day to get the hang of it. The idea is simple. While you are inhaling, contract one muscle group (for example make a fist with your right hand) for five seconds, then exhale and at the same time release the tension in that muscle. As you do so, imagine those stressful feelings flowing out of your body. Then you give yourself a brief break (10–20 seconds), squeeze your eyes shut, and relax, before progressing through these muscle groups: right hand and forearm, right upper arm, left hand and forearm, left upper arm, belly, right thigh, and so on. There are videos at thefast800.com showing you how to do these exercises.

A word of warning, however: you shouldn't think of progressive relaxation as a way of solving your sleep problem. Once you start thinking of it as a solution, like taking a pill, you will start to ask yourself: 'Is it working yet? Do I feel more relaxed? Will I sleep better?' That way madness and insomnia lie.

Mindfulness

My go-to guy for mindfulness is Tim Stead, the author of *See, Love, Be* and a teacher at the world-famous Mindfulness Centre in Oxford. According to Tim, one reason mindfulness can help with sleep problems is that it places a great emphasis on being in the moment; this is important for those of us who spend too much time lying there worrying about what has happened, or fretting about what is going to happen.

To get an impression of what mindfulness entails, try doing this exercise right now: sit up straight, close your eyes and bring your attention to your breath, focusing on your chest rising and your lungs filling as your breath moves in and out of your body. No need to slow it down or speed it up; just see if it is possible to keep your attention on your own breath. If you notice that your mind has wandered, which it will, return to focus on your breathing. Don't dwell on the thoughts, simply notice them and let them drift away, like leaves on a stream.

The art of mindfulness is to keep doing this, but for progressively longer periods of time. If you can manage 10 minutes once a day you will be doing well. Twenty minutes would be better.

Tim says that mindfulness helps because it encourages you to accept that you are awake and that is fine. Once you let go, once you stop worrying about not going to sleep, then sleep will come. Like exercise, mindfulness is not a quick fix and it is unlikely that you will be able to do it successfully on your own. There are apps like Headspace, or Calm, that will guide you, or you could enrol on a mindfulness course.

Recipe suggestions for week 3

- Banana on toast with crunchy walnuts (page 285)
- Super-speedy mushroom risotto with edamame (page 246)
- Cheesy celeriac and anchovy bake (page 261)

BONUS EXERCISE FOR WEEK 3

MICHAEL'S HIIT REGIME

My regime consists of three bursts of 20 seconds, done three times a week on an exercise bike. You should only attempt this once you have built up some fitness. If you are unfit, you should start by doing two lots of 10 seconds, then slowly build your way up over the course of a few weeks.

1. Get on an exercise bike and do a couple of minutes of gentle cycling, against limited resistance, to warm up. You should just about notice the effort in your thighs.
2. After a couple of minutes, begin pedalling fast, then swiftly crank up the resistance. The amount of resistance you select will depend on your strength and fitness. It should be high enough for you to feel it after 15 seconds of sprinting.
3. If, after 15 seconds, you can still keep going at the same pace without too much effort, the resistance you've chosen isn't high enough.

It mustn't, however, be so high that you grind to a complete halt. It's a matter of experimenting. What you'll find is that as you get fitter, the amount of resistance you can cope with increases. It's not speed but effort you are after.

4. After your first burst of fast sprinting, drop the resistance and do a couple of minutes of gentle pedalling to get your breath back.

5. Then do it twice more.

6. Finish with a couple of minutes of gentle cycling to allow your heart rate and blood pressure to return to normal before stepping off the bike. In total, this takes me less than 10 minutes.

Week four

Once again, I hope you are filling in your sleep diary. By now you should definitely be seeing improvements in the quality of your sleep, and you will be finding it easier to fall asleep and stay asleep. You should be feeling less tired during the day, which in turn will motivate you to do more of the exercises that I have been recommending. Here are my suggestions for what to do in week 4 to keep the momentum going and make these sleep techniques a natural, ongoing part of your routine.

MONDAY

If you are doing SRT, things should be getting easier. Once you have built your sleep efficiency back up to 85% and feel you are getting a satisfying, refreshing amount of sleep, then maintain the same bedtime and wake up routine every day. As I mentioned earlier, some people will find that three weeks of SRT is enough to mend their sleep problems, but others will have to keep going.

TUESDAY

Boost your M score further by eating a handful of nuts every day, expanding your seafood repertoire (why not try Clare's Warm salmon and butternut pumpkin salad, page 273) and cutting right back on processed foods (which are usually packed with artificial additives that your gut microbiome doesn't like). Can you go beyond 5-a-day to boost your gut microbiome? The fermented pickled onion you made in the first week of the plan should be ready now, so tuck in!

WEDNESDAY

Get into the habit of avoiding bright lights at night, which could otherwise inhibit the release of melatonin, the hormone of darkness which helps get your brain and body lined up for sleep. Listening to some slow tunes just before bed can also be deeply relaxing; your best bet is classical, jazz or folk music as these are the most effective sleep inducers.

THURSDAY

If you've been comfortably letting breakfast slip later and later in your schedule, see if you can extend your night-time fast to 14 or even 16 hours, to take advantage of the sleep-inducing benefits of TRE. Just make sure lunch is nutritious and protein-rich (try Clare's Black bean salad with lime and avocado, page 252).

FRIDAY

Have you been having a go at mindfulness? Doing a proper course can be demanding, but 'Mindfulness' can be as simple as focusing intently on what's on your fork – the taste, the texture, the smell – or concentrating on your breath as it enters and leaves your body. If you do wake up in the night, mindfulness can help you accept that you are awake without worrying about the possible implications of sleeplessness.

SATURDAY

You're so nearly at the end of your sleep plan! It's time to treat yourself with a celebration dinner (packed with vegetables and pulses, naturally) and a glass of wine if you want to. Just make a point of bringing dinner a little earlier if you can so that you get into the habit of finishing your last meal of the day at least three hours before you go to bed. This gives your body plenty of time to digest and ensures your core body temperature naturally starts to fall as bedtime approaches to help trigger sleep. For optimal sleep (now and in the future) stick to no more than one glass of alcohol a day, ideally red (because it has some health-giving qualities) and only with your evening meal.

SUNDAY

Congratulations! You've made it to the end of the course! By now your sleep quality should be significantly improved to the point where you are sleeping soundly for most of the night, and not worrying unduly if you do wake up. If you're not quite there yet, do continue with the plan and keep following the suggestions.

Life is likely to seem so much sweeter now that you're sleeping well, but don't take good sleep for granted. You could still be vulnerable to falling back into unhelpful old habits. So it's a really good idea to stick to a regular sleep window, going to bed and waking up at the same time seven days a week – weekends included – to follow a healthy

Mediterranean-based diet, and to keep a lid on your stress levels by practising mindfulness and breathing exercises whenever you can.

Some longer-term goals:

LOOKING AFTER YOUR OLD FRIENDS

If you have been eating meals from the recipe section in this book, I would also expect your gut microbiome to have changed radically, and for the better. Your levels of 'good' bacteria should have increased, reducing inflammation and making you feel more cheerful, while the 'bad' ones, that cause inflammation, will have been displaced. So keep munching those legumes! Remember that quite apart from the positive impact that these foods have on your sleep, they will also help cut your risk of type 2 diabetes, heart disease and dementia. Treat this way of eating as a way of life, not just a quick fix when it comes to improving your sleep.

EATING FOR BETTER HEALTH AND WEIGHT LOSS

As we have seen, if you are overweight, even losing a bit of fat will make a huge difference to your sleep and the quality of your life.

At the beginning of the plan, I recommended you write down your weight, waist size, neck size and blood sugar levels. Have they improved?

I wrote that ideally your waist should be less than half your height, and if you are not there yet, are you getting a bit closer? If your neck size has decreased, has that had an effect on your snoring? How about your blood sugar levels? Were they a problem before you started, and if so, have they fallen? If you have blood sugars that put you in the diabetes range, I would strongly recommend you check out thefast800.com website for more information on the benefits of rapid weight loss.

BECOMING MORE ACTIVE

Have you been doing more exercise? I would hope that you have started both the resistance exercises and doing HIIT a few times a week. As your sleep improves, you will find doing exercise much more enjoyable. It really is key to healthy living. Do keep going.

KEEP CALM AND CARRY ON

It is early days, but if you have been practising the breathing and muscle relaxation exercises, you should soon start reaping the benefits.

Mindfulness is demanding, at least initially, and the benefits take longer to become apparent. But if you are stressed and haven't yet decided to give it a go, then I would strongly recommend trying an app or signing up for a course.

Recipe suggestions for week 4

- Mushroom, chickpea and kale curry (page 266)
- Pasta with peas and goat's cheese (page 242)
- Dorset apple cake (page 284)

BONUS EXERCISE FOR WEEK 4

VIGOROUS AEROBIC EXERCISE

The standard recommendations are to do at least 150 minutes of moderate aerobic activity (walking, swimming, mowing the lawn) or 75 minutes of vigorous aerobic activity (running, cycling, dancing) a week. Why not try one you enjoy?

I do a lot of brisk walking (I aim for at least 30 minutes a day) and I also cycle everywhere. There are lots of proven benefits of exercise and strength training (for more on these go to thefast800.com).

I do my HIIT workout at home (page 210), but it is best, at least to start with, to do it in a supervised setting such as a gym. As with any other form of exercise, it would be wise to discuss with your doctor before starting, particularly if you are on medication.

The 4-Week Sleep Plan in brief

WEEK ONE

- Clear out your bedroom and order any equipment or supplements (sleep trackers, light box, melatonin, Bimuno).
- Establish good bedtime habits.
- Start keeping a sleep diary.
- Eat more Mediterranean-style foods.
- If you're going for the sleep reboot, use your sleep diary or tracker to work out your sleep efficiency.
- To reboot your sleep, reduce the amount of time you spend in bed each night so it matches the time you actually spend sleeping each night.
- If you don't think you can handle a full reboot, simply follow the other suggestions in this book and try reducing your sleep window by just one hour.

WEEK TWO

- If your sleep efficiency has improved to 85%, add 20 minutes to your sleep window.
- If you're not seeing any improvement, keep going for another week.
- Incorporate TRE (14:10) into your life.
- Add in some exercise or at least increase your activity levels.

WEEK THREE

- If your sleep efficiency really doesn't improve after two weeks of sleep restriction, cut the time you spend in bed by another 20 minutes. In other words, if you started by spending six hours in bed, you will now have to go down to five hours and 40 minutes. (NB: Never go below five hours in bed).
- Practise challenging your catastrophic thoughts.
- Do breathing and muscle relaxation exercises.

WEEK FOUR

- Your sleep efficiency should by now have improved significantly, and you should be feeling much better during the day. If you feel that you are getting sufficient sleep, then you can ease up on the sleep restriction. If not, keep going.
- Remember to get outside first thing for at least half an hour to soak up the light.
- Keep eating that Mediterranean-style food.
- Continue with the mindfulness, breathing exercises and other forms of stress-busting and relaxation.

Once you have got your insomnia under control the best way to ensure you go on sleeping well is to follow these eight simple rules:

1. Stick to a regular sleep window, i.e. a regular wake-up-go-to-bed routine.
2. Use the sleep tips from Chapter 5 that work for you.

3. Manage your stress levels by trying to practise some mindfulness or breathing exercises during the day.

4. Get out of bed if you can't go to sleep and don't get back in until you feel tired.

5. Expose yourself to bright light (daylight or a light box) first thing in the morning.

6. Remain active and do plenty of resistance exercises like press-ups and squats.

7. Eat a Med-style diet with some fermented foods.

8. Try to keep your belly fat down by aiming for a waist that is less than half your height.

Goodnight from me

Insomnia is a serious condition that affects hundreds of millions of people worldwide. In recent years, there's been mounting concern about the impact that shift work and sleep deprivation have on our brains and bodies. The sleep industry is huge and growing fast, yet few of the things they are selling actually work.

The methods I have outlined in this book, however, do have strong scientific support and I am sure they will help most people who have a sleeping problem. If you have suffered from insomnia for a long time, as I have, it will be harder to crack than if you occasionally have a bad night, but it can be done!

If, despite working on your sleep plan as suggested, you are still struggling, it may be worth discussing it with your GP.

Long-term insomniacs are also at greater risk of being tipped back into their sleepless state by stressful life events. It won't necessarily happen, but if it does, don't worry. Just redo the 4-Week Sleep Plan and in a short while things should once more be under control. Good luck! And do visit my website at thefast800.com for more tips on how to stay healthy.

Recipes

BY DR CLARE BAILEY AND JUSTINE PATTISON

I have been a GP for more than 30 years and over that time I have seen hundreds of patients with sleep problems. I am delighted to say that many report sleeping better when they follow my advice and switch to a moderately low-carb, high-fibre Mediterranean-style diet. This is partly because of the effect it has on their waist and their necks and therefore on how much they snore. But it is also because of something most of them are unaware of: the impact that a change in diet is having on their microbiome.

These recipes have been carefully chosen to help you boost nutrients and increase your fibre intake, all for the benefit of looking after your microbiome so that it looks after you.

Dr Clare Bailey

NB: all calorie counts are for one serving.

Breakfast and brunch

These easy-to-prepare breakfasts are filling and tasty, to help you get going in the morning and keep your energy levels up.

Black grapes with yoghurt and almonds

With a boost of gut-friendly live yoghurt and the anti-inflammatory resveratrol in the grapes, this is a great way to start the day.

Serves 1 – 255 calories

100g full-fat live Greek yoghurt or plant-based yoghurt

50g black or red seedless grapes, halved

10g flaked almonds, toasted

1 tsp runny honey (optional)

1. Spoon the yoghurt into a bowl or glass tumbler. Top with the grapes and flaked almonds, drizzle with honey, if using, and serve.

Cook's tip: If you can't buy ready-toasted almonds, simply toast your own. Scatter the almonds into a dry frying pan and cook for 2–3 minutes over a medium heat, tossing regularly, until lightly browned.

If making as a portable breakfast, assemble the ingredients in a lidded container and keep chilled until you are ready to eat.

Oaty nutty shake

A delicious, creamy porridge shake will help lower your cholesterol, as well as giving you a good portion of healthy nuts.

Serves 2 – 295 calories

40g plain cashew nuts (not roasted)

4 tbsp porridge oats (around 25g)

350ml full-fat milk or plant-based milk

1 tsp maple syrup

¼ tsp ground cinnamon

1. Place the nuts in a bowl and cover with cold water. Refrigerate and leave to soak for 4–6 hours, to soften. If you have a really powerful blender, you can skip the soaking stage.
2. Drain the nuts and place in a jug. Add the oats, milk, maple syrup and cinnamon and blitz with a stick blender until as smooth as possible, adding a little extra milk if needed. (You could do this in a blender or food processor.)
3. Pour into two glass tumblers to serve.

Rosy overnight oats

Oh, the joy of stumbling into the kitchen and being able to dig straight into this creamy, oaty breakfast pot! It's also a great way to get a good dose of fibre.

Serves 2 – 330 calories

1 small apple, quartered, cored and coarsely grated

100g frozen mixed berries or fresh berries in season

50g jumbo porridge oats

25g flaked almonds, toasted

8 ready-to-eat dried apricots, roughly chopped

75g full-fat live Greek yoghurt or plant-based yoghurt

100ml full-fat milk or plant-based milk

1. Place the apple in a large bowl then stir in the frozen berries, oats, almonds, apricots, yoghurt and enough milk to reach a soft, creamy consistency (it will thicken as it stands). Cover and refrigerate for several hours or overnight.

2. To serve, divide into two small bowls (or take to work in lidded pots) and add extra milk, if needed. This will keep well for up to 2 days if chilled.

Cook's tip: If you can't buy ready-toasted almonds see page 225 for a tip on how to toast them.

Scrambled eggs with kimchi

This is Michael's favourite breakfast at the moment – and a great boost to a healthy, sleep-enhancing microbiome.

Serves 2 – 345 calories

15g butter or olive oil

4 large eggs, well beaten

2 slices seeded sourdough (around 40g per slice)

50g kimchi (Korean pickled cabbage – see tip) or sauerkraut

1. Melt the butter or heat the oil in a medium non-stick saucepan.
2. Add the eggs, season with flaked sea salt and freshly ground black pepper and cook over a low heat for 2–3 minutes, stirring regularly, until lightly set.
3. Meanwhile, toast the bread on both sides and divide between two plates. Top with the scrambled eggs and serve with the kimchi or sauerkraut alongside.

Cook's tip: Kimchi is available in most large supermarkets and in health food shops. You could try making it yourself (see recipe in *The Fast 800*, page 241).

Sweet potato savoury muffins with feta

Enjoy as breakfast or brunch with a large salad, either hot from the oven or cold the next day. Keeping the skin on the sweet potato not only saves time peeling, but adds lots of extra nutrients and fibre.

Makes 6 – 335 calories

5 tbsp olive or canola oil, plus extra for greasing

1 sweet potato (around 225g), scrubbed well and cut into roughly
   1cm chunks

1 medium onion, peeled and roughly chopped

1 tbsp fresh thyme leaves (or ½ tsp dried thyme)

100g ground almonds

50g brown self-raising flour

½ tsp baking powder

1 large egg

125ml full-fat milk

100g feta or goat's cheese, cut into roughly 1cm cubes

25g Parmesan, finely grated

1. Preheat the oven to 220°C/fan 200°C/gas 7. Generously grease a 6-hole non-stick muffin tin with oil.
2. Scatter the sweet potato over a small roasting tin. Toss with 1 tablespoon of the oil, season with flaked sea salt and freshly ground black pepper and roast for 10 minutes.
3. Remove from the oven and turn the pieces of sweet potato. Scatter the onion and thyme leaves into the roasting tin and return to

the oven. Roast for a further 15–20 minutes, or until the sweet potato and onion are tender and lightly browned. Meanwhile, place the ground almonds, flour and baking powder in a bowl and whisk in the remaining oil, egg and milk.

4. Stir the roasted vegetables into the batter and divide between the holes of the muffin tin. Dot with the pieces of feta or goat's cheese and sprinkle with the grated Parmesan. Bake for 20–25 minutes, or until puffed up and golden brown. Eat warm or cold.

Cook's tip: If your muffin tin is losing its non-stick properties, line with circles of baking parchment.

Light meals

Most of these easy meals are low in calories, as well as being quick and easy to prepare. Perfect for a light lunch with lots of fibre for those microbes to chomp on.

Cauliflower and roasted red capsicum soup

A creamy soup, full of soluble fibre and with loads of flavour. For a more filling meal, serve the soup topped with crumbled blue cheese or scattered with toasted seeds.

Serves 5–6 – 120 calories

3 tbsp extra-virgin olive oil

1 large onion, peeled and roughly chopped

4 celery sticks, trimmed and thinly sliced

1 garlic clove, peeled and thinly sliced

1 medium cauliflower, trimmed and cut into roughly 3cm chunks, including the stem (roughly 450g prepared weight)

175g roasted red capsicums from a jar, drained

1.5 litres chicken or vegetable stock (fresh or made with 1½ stock cubes)

handful fresh parsley or coriander, leaves roughly chopped, to serve
(optional)

1. Heat the oil in a large saucepan and gently fry the onion and celery for 5 minutes, or until softened and beginning to brown, stirring regularly. Add the garlic and cook for a few seconds more, stirring constantly.

2. Add the cauliflower, red capsicums and stock to the pan and bring to the boil. Reduce the heat, cover loosely with a lid and simmer for about 20 minutes, or until the cauliflower is soft, stirring occasionally. Remove the pan from the heat and blitz with a stick blender until smooth. (You could do this in a food processor.)

3. Season with flaked sea salt and lots of freshly ground black pepper to taste. Warm through gently, stirring regularly, adding a little extra water, if needed, then ladle into warmed bowls to serve. Sprinkle with parsley or coriander, if using.

Jerusalem artichoke soup

A perfect way to enjoy one of the ultimate, sleep-enhancing, high-fibre vegetables. Keep the skin on to retain all the best nutrients. If you aren't used to Jerusalem artichokes, serve small portions to begin with as increasing fibre may create wind at first.

Serves 4 – 325 calories

4 tbsp extra-virgin olive oil
2 medium onions, peeled and finely chopped

2 garlic cloves, peeled and crushed

800g Jerusalem artichokes, scrubbed well and cut into roughly
   1cm slices

750ml chicken or vegetable stock (fresh or made with 1 stock cube)

4 tbsp mixed seeds (around 40g), ideally toasted

1. Heat the oil in a large saucepan. Add the onions, garlic and artichokes, cover with a lid and cook gently for 15 minutes, or until the vegetables are very soft, stirring occasionally.

2. Add the stock and bring to a simmer. Cook uncovered for 5 minutes, stirring regularly.

3. Remove the pan from the heat and blitz with a stick blender until smooth. (You could do this in a food processor.)

4. Season with flaked sea salt and freshly ground black pepper to taste, then warm through gently. Ladle the soup into warmed bowls and serve in small portions, sprinkled with the seeds.

Cook's tip: Toast the mixed seeds in a dry frying pan over a low heat for 2–3 minutes, or until just coloured, stirring constantly. For a richer-tasting soup, add a little full-fat milk or cream when reheating.

This soup freezes beautifully so, if you don't think you'll get through it all in a couple of days, pop the rest into the freezer.

Anti-inflammatory Chinese-style chicken broth

This is a gut-soothing chicken broth, full of vital nutrients. You can enjoy it as a clear soup or see page 234 for a fuller version with added fibre, veg and protein.

Serves 4 (makes 1.5 litres) – 170 calories

500g organic chicken wings and/or leftover roasted chicken

1 onion, peeled and quartered

1 medium carrot, well scrubbed, trimmed and sliced

2 celery sticks, trimmed and cut into roughly 2cm lengths

4 garlic cloves, peeled and halved

50g piece fresh root ginger, peeled and thinly sliced

½ tsp Chinese five-spice powder

1. Place the chicken wings in a large saucepan with the onion, carrot, celery, garlic, ginger and five-spice powder. (If using leftover roast chicken, discard any skin and take any meat off the bones, refrigerate in a covered bowl. Place the remaining carcass in the saucepan.) Pour over 2 litres cold water to cover all the ingredients and cover with a lid.

2. Place over the heat and bring to a very gentle simmer (the water should be barely bubbling) and cook for at least 4 hours, but up to 6 hours if you have the time. Skim off any foam that rises to the surface and top up the water, if needed.

3. Ladle the stock through a fine sieve into a large bowl or saucepan. Save any usable pieces of chicken meat from the bones and

discard the rest. Serve the broth with the reserved meat, use as stock or cool completely before covering and placing in the fridge or freezer.

Cook's tip: You can prepare the stock in a slow cooker for several hours or overnight. Refer to the manufacturer's guidelines for correct quantities of water for the best results.

Chicken noodles with pak choi

Pak choi is an excellent source of soluble fibre, as are mushrooms and spring onions. We love this as a quick and easy light lunch – reminiscent of food from stalls in South East Asia.

Serves 4 – 245 calories

1.5 litres Anti-inflammatory Chinese-style chicken broth (see page
   233) or 1.5 litres water and 1½ chicken or vegetable stock cubes
150g dried wholewheat or buckwheat noodles
150g mushrooms (any kind but shiitake are particularly good), sliced
100–200g cooked chicken
4 spring onions, trimmed and sliced
4 small pak choi, trimmed and thickly sliced
1 tbsp sesame oil
1 long red chilli, thinly sliced, or ½ tsp crushed dried chilli flakes
   (optional)
1–1½ tbsp dark soy sauce, to taste

1. Pour the stock into a large saucepan and add the noodles, mushrooms, cooked chicken, spring onions, pak choi, sesame oil and chilli, if using. Bring to a gentle simmer and cook for 3 minutes, or until the noodles are soft.
2. Season with soy sauce to serve.

Tofu, leek and kimchi broth

A lovely, exotic, Korean-inspired noodle soup that includes the benefits of fermented kimchi.

Serves 2 – 320 calories

1 tbsp sesame oil

1 medium leek, trimmed and thinly sliced

2 garlic cloves, peeled and crushed

50g kimchi

100g dried wholewheat or soba noodles

500ml hot vegetable or chicken stock (for fresh, see page 233; or
    make it with boiling water and 1 stock cube)

150g soft silken tofu, cut into roughly 2cm cubes

2 spring onions, trimmed and thinly sliced

1 red chilli, trimmed and thinly sliced

handful fresh coriander, leaves roughly chopped, to serve

soy sauce, to taste

1. Heat the oil in a saucepan and fry the leek for 3 minutes, or until soft. Add the garlic and kimchi and cook for 1 further minute, stirring.

2. Meanwhile, cook the noodles for 3–4 minutes, or according to the packet instructions.

3. Pour the stock into the pan with the leek mixture and bring to a simmer. Add the tofu, spring onions and chilli and cook for 3 minutes, stirring once.

4. Drain the noodles and divide between two wide bowls. Spoon the broth on top, sprinkle with fresh coriander and add soy sauce to taste.

Curried lentil soup with turmeric

This rich, tasty soup offers gut-friendly fibre in the lentils along with the gorgeous golden glow of turmeric. Turmeric's anti-inflammatory health benefits are enhanced by combining it with coconut oil and black pepper.

Serves 4 – 580 calories

2 tbsp olive or canola oil

1 onion, peeled and finely chopped

1 tbsp medium curry powder

2 tsp ground turmeric

25g piece fresh root ginger, peeled and finely chopped

200g dried red split lentils

1 × 400ml can full-fat organic coconut milk

juice 1 lime or ½ lemon

handful fresh coriander, leaves roughly chopped, to serve

For the crispy fried onions:

6 tbsp olive or canola oil

1 onion, peeled and sliced into thin rings

1. To make the soup, heat the oil in a large saucepan and gently fry the onion for 5 minutes, or until softened, stirring regularly. Add the curry powder, turmeric and ginger and cook for 1 further minute, stirring.

2. Add the lentils, coconut milk and 800ml cold water. Bring to a gentle simmer, partially cover with a lid and cook for 20–25 minutes, or until the lentils are very soft, stirring more frequently towards the end of the cooking time. Add a little extra water if needed.

3. Just before the soup is ready, prepare the crispy onions. Place the oil in a small saucepan over a medium heat. Add the onion and fry for 6 minutes, or until golden and crisp, stirring frequently. Take off the heat, remove the onion with a slotted spoon and drain on kitchen paper.

4. Add the lemon or lime juice to the soup and season with flaked sea salt and freshly ground black pepper, to taste. Ladle into warmed bowls and top with golden onion rings and coriander.

Cook's tip: To turn this recipe into a lentil dahl for a more substantial meal, cook with around 600ml water instead and top with halved hard-boiled eggs as well as the onion rings.

If making ahead, you may need to add extra water when reheating.

Baked chicory with prosciutto

Chicory roots are one of the best sources of soluble fibre, supporting gut health and, by association, boosting mood. A light, flavoursome dish.

Serves 2 – 395 calories

1 tbsp extra-virgin olive oil, plus extra for greasing

2 large heads chicory (each around 150g)

4 thin slices prosciutto or Parma ham (around 55g total weight)

40g walnut halves, roughly chopped

25g Parmesan, finely grated

2 tsp cider or white wine vinegar, or lemon juice

1. Preheat the oven to 200°C/fan 180°C/gas 6. Lightly oil a small baking tray.
2. Trim a slim sliver off the base of each head of chicory and cut in half lengthwise. Place cut side down on the baking tray and bake for 18–20 minutes, or until just tender.
3. Take the tray out of the oven, turn the chicory over and drizzle with the oil. Drape the prosciutto over the top and sprinkle with the walnuts and Parmesan. Bake for a further 5–8 minutes, or until the walnuts are lightly toasted and the Parmesan is melted and beginning to brown.
4. Divide between two warmed plates, drizzle with the vinegar or lemon juice, season generously with freshly ground black pepper and serve.

Dr Tim's hot-smoked salmon salad

This delicious salad is so easy to make even Dr Tim can do it. And it's super healthy, too.

Serves 2 – 630 calories

150g frozen edamame beans or baby broad beans

150g broccoli, cut into small florets

150g hot-smoked salmon or smoked mackerel fillets, flaked

50g young spinach leaves (roughly 2 handfuls)

1 small ripe avocado, stoned, peeled and sliced

¼–½ tsp crushed dried chilli flakes or 1 red chilli, finely sliced (optional)

25g flaked almonds, toasted

juice of ½ lemon

2 tbsp extra-virgin olive oil

1. Third fill a saucepan with water and bring to the boil. Add the frozen edamame or broad beans and broccoli and return to the boil. Cook for 3 minutes, then tip into a colander to drain and rinse under running water until cold.
2. Place the vegetables in a large serving bowl and add the salmon or mackerel, spinach, avocado and chilli, if using. Toss together lightly.
3. Sprinkle with the almonds, drizzle with the lemon juice and olive oil, season with freshly ground black pepper and serve.

Baked sweet potato with smoked mackerel

A tasty way to up your omega-3 intake.

Serves 2 – 630 calories

2 medium-large sweet potatoes (each around 250g), scrubbed well

2 smoked mackerel fillets (each around 75g), skinned

10 cherry tomatoes, quartered

¼ cucumber, cut into roughly 1cm chunks

2 tbsp good-quality mayonnaise

4 tbsp full-fat live Greek yoghurt

4–6 radishes, finely sliced, or Purple pickled onions (see page 290), to
serve (optional)

1. Preheat the oven to 200°C/fan 180°C/gas 6.
2. Place the sweet potatoes on a baking tray and prick each one a couple of times with a fork. Bake for 50–60 minutes, or until tender.
3. Just before the potatoes are ready, flake the mackerel fillets into a bowl and add the tomatoes, cucumber, mayonnaise and yoghurt. Season with freshly ground black pepper and mash together roughly.
4. Divide the sweet potatoes between two plates and make a cross in the middle of each one. Open out, stuff with the mackerel mixture, top with the radishes and serve.

Cook's tip: You could also cook the sweet potatoes in the microwave – for around 8 minutes on high.

Griddled eggplant with feta and pine nuts

Luscious dark eggplant is the star of this dish, delivering plenty of fibre and antioxidants to help get your gut into top condition. Some research even suggests it helps lower blood sugars.

Serves 2 – 375 calories

½ tsp ground cumin

½ tsp ground coriander

3 tbsp extra-virgin olive oil

1 medium-large eggplant (around 300g), trimmed and sliced into
   6 lengthwise

2 tbsp pine nuts (around 20g)

100g feta, roughly cubed

large pinch crushed dried chilli flakes (optional)

10g fresh coriander, leaves roughly chopped

juice ½ lemon

1. Preheat a large griddle pan until hot.
2. Mix the cumin and coriander in a small bowl with a good pinch flaked sea salt and lots of freshly ground black pepper. Add 2 table-spoons of the oil and stir well. Brush the eggplant slices on both sides with the seasoned oil.
3. Place the eggplant slices on the griddle pan and cook, in batches if necessary, for 4–5 minutes, or until lightly browned. Then turn and cook on the other side for a further 4–5 minutes, until

browned and very tender. (If cooking in batches, keep the first batch warm in the oven while the second batch is cooking.)

4. While the eggplant is cooking, toast the pine nuts in a small dry frying pan over a medium heat for 2–3 minutes, or until lightly browned, stirring regularly.

5. Divide the eggplant slices between two plates and top with the feta. Sprinkle with the pine nuts and chilli flakes, if using. Scatter over the coriander and drizzle with the remaining oil and the lemon juice. Season with more freshly ground black pepper to serve.

Cook's tip: If you don't have a griddle pan, use a large non-stick frying pan. The eggplant slices won't have the griddle stripes but will still taste delicious.

You can add a handful of baby spinach or rocket for extra greens, if you like.

Pasta with peas and goat's cheese

Tasty and very easy to put together, this is made with ingredients you may already have stashed in the freezer or store cupboard, making it a great last-minute meal.

Serves 2 – 625 calories

80g wholewheat pasta, such as penne or fusilli

2 tbsp pine nuts (about 20g)

3 tbsp extra-virgin olive oil

½ small onion, peeled and very finely chopped

1 small garlic clove, peeled and crushed

200g frozen petits pois (or peas)

finely grated zest ½ lemon and 1 tbsp juice

100g goat's cheese, rind removed

1. Half fill a saucepan with water and bring to the boil. Add the pasta and cook for 10–12 minutes, or according to the packet instructions, until just tender, stirring occasionally.

2. Meanwhile, lightly toast the pine nuts in a dry frying pan over a medium heat for 2–3 minutes, or until lightly browned, stirring regularly. Tip on to a plate and set aside.

3. Return the frying pan to the hob and add the oil and onion. Fry over a low heat for 5 minutes, or until softened, stirring regularly. Add the garlic and peas and cook for a further minute, stirring.

4. Drain the pasta and return to the saucepan. Add the fried onion and pea mixture and stir in the lemon zest and juice and the goat's cheese. Toss together over a low heat until the cheese warms and begins to melt.

5. Season with flaked sea salt and freshly ground black pepper and divide between two warmed bowls. Top with the toasted pine nuts to serve.

Hot-smoked salmon, anchovies, artichoke and broccoli pasta

Omega-3 from the oily fish, lots of lovely fibre, as well as nutrient-rich fermented crème fraîche. All you need to soothe you to sleep.

Serves 2 – 610 calories

80g wholewheat pasta, such as penne

1 small head broccoli (around 200g), cut into small florets

4 anchovies in olive oil, from a jar or can, drained and chopped

3 tbsp extra-virgin olive oil

1 small garlic clove, peeled and crushed

1 small sprig fresh rosemary, leaves picked and finely chopped

150g hot-smoked salmon

75g artichoke hearts, from a jar or can, drained and cut into chunks

3 tbsp full-fat crème fraîche

small bunch fresh parsley, leaves roughly chopped

good pinch crushed dried chilli flakes (optional)

1. Half fill a saucepan with water and bring to the boil. Add the pasta and cook for 10 minutes, or according to the packet instructions, until just tender. Add the broccoli to the pasta for the last 3 minutes of the cooking time.

2. Drain the pasta and broccoli, return to the pan and cover loosely with a lid. Place the anchovies, olive oil, garlic and rosemary in a large non-stick frying pan and cook over a low heat for 1 minute, stirring until the anchovies soften and almost dissolve into the oil.

3. Add the salmon and artichoke hearts and heat through gently for 2–3 minutes, stirring gently until hot. Try not to let the salmon break up too much.

4. Tip the pasta and broccoli into the frying pan, add the crème fraîche, parsley and chilli, if using. Season with freshly ground black pepper and toss together gently. Divide between two warm bowls to serve.

Sardines on seeded sourdough

Brain power on toast, with omega-3 to oil those cogs.

Serves 2 – 310 calories

1 × 120g can sardines in olive oil

juice ½ small lemon (around 1 tbsp)

2 thin slices seeded sourdough (each around 40g)

¼ small red onion, peeled and very thinly sliced

1 tsp baby capers, drained (optional)

1 tbsp extra-virgin olive oil

1. Roughly mash the sardines in their oil with the lemon juice, a little flaked sea salt and plenty of freshly ground black pepper.

2. Toast the bread and divide between two plates – or serve for one if you are especially hungry.

3. Spread the mashed sardines on to the hot toast and top with the sliced red onion, capers, if using, and a drizzle of extra-virgin olive oil. Serve immediately, before the toast has time to cool.

Super-speedy mushroom risotto with edamame

Risotto doesn't have to take hours – this lovely mushroom recipe can be made in 15 minutes and is packed with gut-friendly ingredients.

Serves 2 – 410 calories

10g dried porcini mushrooms (or any dried wild mushrooms)

2 tbsp olive oil

1 small onion, peeled and finely chopped

100g chestnut mushrooms, sliced

1 garlic clove, peeled and crushed

250g cooked brown, or mixed brown and wild rice

80g frozen edamame beans

1 tbsp chia seeds

pinch dried thyme

200ml chicken or vegetable stock (fresh or made with ½ stock cube)

30g Parmesan, finely grated

pinch crushed dried chilli flakes (optional)

1. Place the dried mushrooms in a heatproof bowl and cover with 150ml just-boiled water. Leave to stand for about 10 minutes to soften, then strain through a sieve, reserving the soaking liquor.
2. Meanwhile, heat the oil in a large non-stick saucepan and gently fry the onion for 3–4 minutes, or until softened, stirring regularly. Add the chestnut mushrooms, increase the heat, and cook for 2–3 minutes more, or until the mushrooms are lightly browned.

3. Add the garlic and cook for a few seconds before stirring in the soaked porcini (roughly chopping any particularly large ones), along with the liquor.

4. Add the rice, edamame beans, chia seeds and thyme and stir for 1 minute.

5. Pour in the stock and bring to a gentle simmer. Cook for 3 minutes, stirring regularly.

6. Stir in half the Parmesan and season with flaked sea salt, freshly ground black pepper and chilli flakes, if using. Spoon into warmed shallow bowls and sprinkle with the remaining Parmesan to serve.

Cook's tip: You could use pre-cooked brown/wild rice from a packet but make sure it doesn't contain any flavourings or added ingredients (except for a little oil, which is used to keep the grains separate). If you are cooking rice especially for this recipe, you will need around 85g dried mixed brown and wild rice to yield around 250g cooked rice.

If you can't get hold of edamame beans, use frozen peas or broad beans instead.

On the move

It's challenging to eat healthy meals when you are out and about, particularly if you are a shift worker looking for food outside normal working hours. Being prepared will help ensure that you have the right foods to hand and are not dependent on unhealthy snacks from vending machines or petrol stations. There are some great recipes here, which are both portable and nutritious.

Celery with blue cheese dip

Celery may contain lots of water, but it also has plenty of gut-friendly fibre, both soluble and insoluble, while blue cheese adds a rich, tangy flavour to the dip, as well as a dose of healthy microbes. This is also yummy served on wholegrain seeded crackers.

Serves 2 – 225 calories

50g blue cheese, such as Roquefort

50g full-fat live Greek yoghurt

50g full-fat crème fraîche

celery sticks or other vegetable crudités, to serve

1. Place the cheese, yoghurt and crème fraîche in a bowl and mash with a fork until thoroughly combined. Season to taste with freshly ground black pepper.
2. Spoon into a small dish, or lidded container if taking as a packed lunch, and serve with celery sticks for dipping.

Cashew, ricotta and red capsicum dip

A tangy and tasty dip with extra nutrients and creaminess from the cashews.

Serves 4 – 230 calories

100g plain cashew nuts (not roasted)

1 small garlic clove, peeled and roughly chopped

75g roasted red capsicums from a jar, drained

100g ricotta cheese

4 tbsp extra-virgin olive oil, plus extra for drizzling

finely grated zest ½ small lemon

pinch paprika, to serve (optional)

1. Place the nuts in a bowl and pour over just enough cold water to cover. Refrigerate and leave to soak for 4–6 hours, to soften.
2. Drain the nuts and place in a food processor with the garlic, capsicums, ricotta, oil and lemon zest. Blitz until thoroughly combined. Season with flaked sea salt and freshly ground black pepper.

3. Spoon into a serving dish, drizzle with a little oil and sprinkle with paprika, if using. Serve with lots of vegetable sticks or sourdough crispbread.

Cook's tip: If you don't have a food processor, place the soaked cashews and all the remaining ingredients in a bowl or jug and blitz with a stick blender instead. You could use home-roasted red capsicums, instead of the jarred kind, if you like.

Prawns and red cabbage slaw on sourdough

Prawns and slaw on sourdough is an all-round, gut-friendly winner. Sourdough is one of the healthiest breads available, made using a slow process of fermentation, so it is easier to digest and less likely to cause a spike in blood sugar. Michael and I are big fans, and love the flavour and firm texture.

Serves 2 – 270 calories

100g red cabbage, trimmed and very finely sliced

1 small carrot, scrubbed well and coarsely grated

1 tbsp mixed seeds

2 slices sourdough bread (around 40g each slice)

small handful fresh watercress or mixed baby salad leaves (around 20g)

75g cooked and peeled prawns, thawed if frozen and drained

For the dressing:

2 tbsp extra-virgin olive oil

1 tsp fresh lemon juice, plus extra to serve

½ tsp Dijon mustard

½ tsp runny honey (optional)

1. To make the dressing, whisk together the olive oil, lemon juice, mustard and honey in a large bowl.
2. Add the cabbage, carrot and mixed seeds to the bowl with the dressing and toss together.
3. Divide the sourdough between two plates and top with the watercress or salad leaves. Place some red cabbage slaw on top, then scatter over the prawns. Squeeze over a little extra lemon juice and season with freshly ground black pepper to serve.

Smoked mackerel, beetroot and tahini pitta

Juicy, filling and full of flavour, this is a nutritious instant meal. Oily fish has been found not only to improve sleep, but also to improve function during the day.

Serves 1 – 635 calories

1 brown pitta bread

small handful fresh watercress or mixed baby salad leaves

1 fillet smoked mackerel (around 75g), skin removed

1 cooked beetroot (around 40g), sliced

For the dressing:

1 tbsp tahini

2 tbsp full-fat live Greek yoghurt

1 tbsp extra-virgin olive oil

1–2 tsp fresh lemon juice

1. To make the dressing, thoroughly mix the tahini, yoghurt, olive oil and lemon juice with 4 tablespoons cold water in a small bowl. Season with flaked sea salt and freshly ground black pepper.
2. Warm the pitta, if possible, then split open and fill with the watercress or salad leaves. Flake the mackerel into the pitta and add the sliced beetroot. Season with plenty of freshly ground black pepper and drizzle with a little of the dressing.

Cook's tip: The rest of the dressing can be kept in the fridge and used on salads or as a dip for up to 2 days.

Black bean salad with lime and avocado

A tangy and filling salad. The tasty black beans are not only a boost of fibre but also add a generous number of anti-inflammatory phytonutrients and B vitamins, including folate.

Serves 2 – 315 calories

1 × 400g can black beans, drained and rinsed

½ tsp flaked sea salt

100g mangetout or fine green beans, trimmed

1 small ripe but firm avocado, peeled, stoned and sliced

2 spring onions, trimmed and finely sliced

1 red chilli, finely chopped, or ½ tsp crushed dried chilli flakes

20g fresh coriander, leaves roughly chopped

For the lime and sesame dressing:

2 tbsp extra-virgin olive oil

1½ tbsp fresh lime juice

1 tbsp sesame seeds (around 10g), toasted

1. Place the black beans in a serving bowl and toss with the salt. Leave to stand.
2. Third fill a saucepan with water and bring to the boil. Add the mangetout and cook for 2 minutes, until tender but crisp. (If using fine green beans, cook for 3 minutes.) Drain then rinse under running water until cold. Drain again.
3. Tip the mangetout or green beans into the bowl with the black beans and add the avocado, spring onions, chilli and coriander. To make the dressing, whisk the olive oil, lime juice and sesame seeds together in a small bowl and season with lots of freshly ground black pepper. Drizzle the dressing over the salad to serve.

Cook's tip: To toast the sesame seeds, sprinkle into a dry frying pan and place over a medium heat. Stir constantly for 1–2 minutes, until lightly browned. Remove from the heat and tip into a small bowl so they don't continue to brown.

Nori rolled crab

The extra omega-3 in the seaweed, along with the crab, make this nori roll both super-tasty and super-healthy for your gut.

Serves 2 – 420 calories

½ medium avocado, peeled and stoned

100g cooked crabmeat, fresh or canned, drained

1 tbsp fresh lime juice

2 sheets dried nori (20cm square each)

150g cooked and cooled brown rice

For the dip:

2 tbsp dark soy sauce

¼ tsp crushed dried chilli flakes or a dash of sriracha chilli sauce

1 tsp sesame oil

1. Place the avocado on a plate and mash well with a fork.
2. Place the crab in a separate bowl and roughly mash with the lime juice and a good grinding of black pepper.
3. Place one of the nori sheets on a board, shiny side down, and spread half of the avocado evenly over the bottom half of the sheet.
4. Top the avocado with half the rice and press down lightly with the back of a spoon. Spread half the crab mixture in a horizontal line across the centre of the rice.
5. Roll the nori from the bottom up around the filling firmly, using two hands. Seal the edge by brushing with a little water and trim

the edges. Cut the roll into six pieces. Repeat with the remaining nori and filling.

6. Mix the soy sauce, chilli flakes or sriracha and sesame oil in a small bowl and serve alongside as a dip.

Cook's tip: You can use leftover rice for this recipe – as long as it was cooked and then cooled straight away – or boil 50g brown rice according to the packet instructions until tender, then rinse under cold running water and drain well. You should find that 50g dried rice will give you 150g cooked.

Nori chilli popcorn

These are heathy nibbles with an omega-3 boost and an irresistible umami flavour.

Serves 2 – 125 calories

20ml extra-virgin olive oil

30g popping corn

For the nori chilli seasoning:

¼ tsp flaked sea salt

½ sheet nori, torn into roughly 3cm strips

½ tsp crushed dried chilli flakes

1. To make the nori chilli seasoning, place the salt, nori and chilli in a large jug and blitz with a stick blender until very finely chopped but not too powdery.

2. Place 1 teaspoon of the oil in a large saucepan with the corn and stir lightly. Cover the pan with a tight-fitting lid and place over a medium heat. As soon as you hear the corn popping, gently shake the pan forward and backwards – don't be tempted to take off the lid – and continue cooking for about 4 minutes, or until the corn has stopped popping, shaking the pan regularly while holding the lid firmly in place.

3. Remove the pan from the heat and drizzle with the remaining oil. Toss well, then add the nori seasoning and toss again. Tip into a large bowl to serve, discarding any kernels that haven't popped.

Tabbouleh with goat's cheese

Bulgur wheat is a delicious nutty grain, often used to make tabbouleh with chopped salad and herbs. In this recipe, topped with cheese and a tangy garlic dressing, it makes an ideal light and portable meal. Add leftover cold meats, falafel or nuts to make a more filling dish.

Serves 4 – 365 calories

200g bulgur wheat (ideally wholegrain)

½ red onion, peeled and very finely sliced

25g fresh mint, leaves roughly chopped

25g fresh flat-leaf parsley, leaves roughly chopped

50g young spinach leaves

100g goat's cheese, cut into small chunks

2 tbsp mixed seeds

For the dressing:

2 garlic cloves, peeled and crushed

2 tbsp fresh lemon juice

4 tbsp extra-virgin olive oil

1. Half fill a medium saucepan with water, add the bulgur wheat, return to the boil and cook for 10 minutes, or until almost tender, stirring occasionally. Drain in a sieve and rinse well under running water until cold. Drain again thoroughly and tip into a large serving bowl.
2. Add the onion, herbs and spinach to the bowl and season with a good pinch of flaked sea salt and plenty of freshly ground black pepper. Toss together well.
3. To make the dressing, whisk the garlic, lemon juice and olive oil in a small bowl until well combined. Pour over the salad and toss lightly.
4. Scatter the goat's cheese and seeds over the top to serve.

Cook's tip: You can use any cheese you like for this recipe, or you can leave it out altogether. Serve the tabbouleh as an accompaniment to grilled meat, fish or roasted wedges of butternut pumpkin or beetroot.

Main meals

These are more substantial dishes, still based on a Mediterranean-style way of eating, with extra beans, lentils and other good sources of fibre, to help boost your microbiome and enhance your sleep.

Trout with celeriac mash

You just can't beat fresh fish with lemon and a crunchy, nutty topping. This comes with creamy celeriac mash and we recommend only minimal peeling so that you get the benefit of all those extra nutrients found in the skin. Serve with some freshly cooked green vegetables.

Serves 2 – 555 calories

2 rainbow trout or fresh mackerel (each around 270g), cleaned

1 small lemon, thinly sliced

2 tbsp extra-virgin olive oil

40g blanched hazelnuts, roughly chopped

For the mash:

300g celeriac, well scrubbed and gnarled bits removed, cut into
    roughly 2cm chunks

50g full-fat crème fraîche

1. Preheat the oven to 200°C/fan 180°C/gas 6. Line a baking tray
   with non-stick baking paper.
2. Place the trout or mackerel on the tray and insert half the lemon
   slices into each one. Drizzle half a tablespoon of oil over each fish
   and season with freshly ground black pepper. Bake uncovered for
   15 minutes. Remove from the oven and scatter with the hazelnuts
   and cook for a further 5 minutes, or until the hazelnuts are lightly
   toasted.
3. Meanwhile, place the celeriac in a saucepan and cover with cold
   water. Bring to the boil and cook for 10 minutes, or until very soft.
   Drain, then return to the pan.
4. Add the crème fraîche, a little flaked sea salt and lots of freshly
   ground black pepper to the pan and blitz with a stick blender until
   smooth.
5. Divide the mash between two warmed plates, add the fish and
   spoon any loose hazelnuts over the top. Drizzle with the remaining
   oil and serve.

Beef and Jerusalem artichoke casserole

The knobbly Jerusalem artichoke offers masses of gut-friendly insoluble and soluble fibre, and has a lovely, nutty and slightly sweet taste. Serve with some celeriac mash (see recipe on page 259, which should be doubled for four people – add 130 cals per portion) and lots of green leafy vegetables.

Serves 4 – 320 calories

500g braising or stewing beef steak, trimmed and cut into roughly 2.5cm chunks

3 tbsp olive oil

1 onion, peeled and thinly sliced

2 celery sticks, cut into roughly 1.5cm slices

3 medium carrots, trimmed, scrubbed well and cut into roughly 2cm chunks

300g Jerusalem artichokes, scrubbed very well and cut into roughly 2cm chunks

1 beef stock cube

2 tbsp tomato purée

1 tsp dried mixed herbs

1. Preheat the oven to 170°C/fan 150°C/gas 3. Season the beef all over with flaked sea salt and freshly ground black pepper.
2. Heat 1 tablespoon of the oil in a large non-stick frying pan and fry the beef in two batches over a medium-high heat for 2–3 minutes, or until browned, adding a little more oil if needed. Transfer to a flame-proof casserole dish.

3. Add the remaining oil to the frying pan and cook the onion, celery, carrots and artichokes for 6–8 minutes, or until lightly browned, stirring regularly. Tip into the dish with the beef.

4. Pour 100ml just-boiled water into the frying pan and scrape the base of the pan with a wooden spoon to dissolve the bits stuck to the bottom. Pour into the casserole with the beef and veg. Add the stock cube, tomato purée and a further 350ml just-boiled water. Sprinkle with the herbs and bring to a simmer, stirring occasionally. Cover with a lid and cook in the oven for about 2 hours, or until the beef is very tender.

Cheesy celeriac and anchovy bake

The taste of the celeriac is wonderfully enhanced by the anchovies and the health benefits of the dish are boosted by the oily fish. Serve this with spring greens, kale or cavolo nero.

Serves 2 – 420 calories

1 small onion, peeled and sliced

1 tbsp olive oil

400g celeriac, scrubbed and gnarled bits removed, cut in half and then into slices roughly 3mm thick

8 anchovies in olive oil (from a jar or can), drained

30g Gouda or Cheddar (or a mixture), coarsely grated

5 tbsp full-fat crème fraîche

4 tbsp full-fat milk

30g Parmesan, finely grated

1 tsp finely chopped fresh rosemary

1. Preheat the oven to 200°C/fan 180°C/gas 6.
2. Scatter the onion over the base of an ovenproof dish, drizzle with the olive oil and season with a little flaked sea salt and freshly ground black pepper. Arrange the slices of celeriac on top. It should be 3–4 layers deep. Place the anchovies on top, then scatter with the Gouda or Cheddar.
3. Mix the crème fraîche with the milk until it is a pouring consistency, then spoon over the celeriac. Season with more freshly ground black pepper. Cover the dish loosely with foil and bake in the centre of the oven for 55–60 minutes, or until the celeriac is just tender. Remove from the oven and discard the foil. Scatter over the Parmesan and rosemary, then return to the oven for about 10 minutes, or until pale golden brown.

Chicken and veg tray bake

An easy, all-in-one, gut-friendly dish. Serve with a crisp green salad.

Serves 4 – 530 calories (without chorizo)

2 medium red onions, peeled and cut into 8 wedges

300g sweet potatoes, scrubbed and cut into roughly 3cm chunks

300g Jerusalem artichokes (or 150g sweet potato and an extra capsicum), scrubbed and cut into 3cm chunks

2 capsicums (one red and one yellow), deseeded and cut into
   roughly 3cm chunks

50g chorizo, cut into roughly 1cm chunks (optional)

4 large tomatoes (around 475g), quartered

4 tbsp extra-virgin olive oil

4 bone-in, skin-on, free-range chicken thighs (around 730g total weight)

1. Preheat the oven to 200°C/fan 180°C/gas 6.
2. Place the onions, sweet potatoes, artichokes, capsicums, chorizo, if using, and tomatoes in a large deep roasting tin. Drizzle with 1 tablespoon of the oil and toss together lightly.
3. Nestle the chicken thighs among the vegetables, skin-side up. Drizzle with the remaining oil and season with sea salt and ground black pepper. Roast for 45–55 minutes, or until the chicken is thoroughly cooked and the veg is lightly browned.

Chicken tagine with chickpeas and dates

For this fabulous tagine, simply throw in most of the ingredients and let the meat soften and the flavours develop. Serve with quinoa or bulgur wheat and a generous pile of green vegetables.

Serves 4 – 540 calories

4 tbsp extra-virgin olive oil

1 large onion, peeled and thinly sliced

2 garlic cloves, peeled and crushed

2 tbsp harissa paste

8 boneless, skinless chicken thighs (around 650g total weight)

2 × 400g cans chopped tomatoes

1 × 400g can organic chickpeas

8 soft pitted dates, thickly sliced

40g blanched almonds (optional)

1 chicken stock cube

20g fresh coriander, stalks finely chopped and leaves coarsely chopped

1. Preheat the oven to 200°C/fan 180°C/gas 6.
2. Heat the oil in a flame-proof casserole and add the onion, garlic and harissa. Stir for 30 seconds to 1 minute over a medium heat. Add the chicken, chopped tomatoes, chickpeas and their water, dates, almonds, stock cube and 100ml water. Season with lots of freshly ground black pepper and a pinch of flaked sea salt.
3. Bring to a gentle simmer, stirring occasionally. Add the chopped coriander stalks, then cover the casserole with a lid and cook in the oven for 1 hour, stirring occasionally, or until the chicken is very tender and the sauce has thickened. Stir half the chopped coriander leaves into the tagine, then sprinkle with the rest just before serving.

Meatballs with feta and eggplant

These meatballs are beautifully complemented by the eggplant, with its an-tioxidants for reducing inflammation. Serve with leafy greens or a salad, and small portions of brown rice or bulgur wheat for a more substantial meal.

Serves 4 – 420 calories

4 tbsp olive oil

20 small ready-made lamb meatballs (around 500g)

1 red onion, peeled and finely chopped

1 eggplant (around 300g), cut into roughly 2cm chunks

1 × 400g can chopped tomatoes

100ml red wine (roughly 1 small glass)

1 tsp dried oregano

½ tsp crushed dried chilli flakes

100g feta

1. Place 1 tablespoon of the oil in a large, deep, non-stick frying pan over a medium heat. Add the meatballs and fry for 8–10 minutes, or until lightly browned on all sides, turning regularly. Transfer the meatballs to a plate and spoon off the excess fat. Return the pan to the heat.

2. Add the remaining oil and fry the onion and eggplant for 6–8 minutes, or until the onion is softened and the eggplant is lightly browned, stirring regularly.

3. Tip the tomatoes into the pan and add the red wine, oregano, chilli and 200ml cold water. Season with flaked sea salt and freshly ground black pepper and bring to a gentle simmer. Return the meatballs to the pan and cook in the sauce for 15 minutes, stirring regularly. Add a splash more water if needed.

4. Finally, crumble the feta over the top and gently simmer without

stirring for a further 3–4 minutes, or until the cheese is hot and has melted slightly into the sauce.

Cook's tip: You can make this recipe using beef meatballs, veggie meatballs or ready-made falafel. If using falafel, serve 2–3 per person and don't pre-fry. Instead, add them to the sauce after it has been simmering for 10 minutes.

Mushroom, chickpea and kale curry

A super-healthy curry – easy, creamy and full of flavour. Serve with brown rice and a tomato and onion salad.

Serves 3 – 580 calories

3 tbsp extra-virgin olive oil

1 onion, peeled and finely chopped

200g small chestnut mushrooms, quartered

2 garlic cloves, peeled and crushed

15g fresh root ginger, peeled and finely chopped

1–1½ tbsp medium curry powder (to taste)

1 × 400ml can full-fat organic coconut milk

150g curly kale, thickly shredded and tough stalks discarded

1 × 400g can organic chickpeas, not drained

40g cashew nuts (not roasted), roughly chopped

squeeze lemon or lime juice (optional)

1. Heat the oil in a large wide-based saucepan or shallow casserole and gently fry the onion for a further 2–3 minutes, stirring regularly. Increase the heat and add the mushrooms and cook for a further 2–3 minutes, or until lightly browned, stirring.

2. Add the garlic, ginger and curry powder and cook for a further 30 seconds, stirring constantly. Pour over the coconut milk and stir in the kale, chickpeas and their water and the cashew nuts. Bring to a simmer, cover with a lid and cook for 10 minutes, or until the kale is tender, stirring occasionally.

3. Season with flaked sea salt and freshly ground pepper to taste, adding a squeeze of lemon or lime juice, if using, to serve.

Cook's tip: Use organic chickpeas in water and you can add them straight from the can. If you can't find organic chickpeas, drain and rinse them instead and add an extra 150ml water to the curry.

Ratatouille with white beans

This works well as a main meal or a side – a glorious, soluble-fibre-rich ratatouille. It is also rich in anti-inflammatory olive oil. This ratatouille can be enjoyed on its own or served alongside fried halloumi, cooked meats or fish.

Serves 2 as a main – 545 calories
(or serves 4 as an accompaniment)

5 tbsp extra-virgin olive oil

2 medium onions, peeled and finely chopped

200g chestnut mushrooms, sliced

1 eggplant (around 350g), cut into roughly 2cm chunks

4 garlic cloves, peeled and crushed

1 tsp dried oregano

1 × 400g can organic white beans, such as cannellini, haricot or
    butter beans

1 × 400g can chopped tomatoes

1 vegetable stock cube

1. Heat 4 tablespoons of the oil in a wide-based saucepan or shallow casserole and gently fry the onions for 6–8 minutes, or until softened, stirring regularly.

2. Add the mushrooms and eggplant, increase the heat, and fry until lightly browned, stirring constantly.

3. Add the garlic and oregano and cook for a few seconds more, stirring.

4. Pour in the beans and their water. Add the tomatoes, crumble over the stock cube and stir 300ml water into the pan. Bring to a gentle simmer, then cover with a lid and cook for 20 minutes. Remove the lid and cook for a further 10 minutes, or until the vegetables are soft and the tomatoes have reduced.

5. Season to taste with flaked sea salt and freshly ground black pepper. Drizzle with the remaining oil to serve.

Shepherd's pie with parsnip and white bean mash

There is lots of glorious fibre in this shepherd's pie, thanks to all the vegetables, lentils and beans. Good, sleep-inducing comfort food. Serve with plenty of freshly cooked green leafy vegetables.

Serves 6 – 355 calories

1 tbsp olive oil

400g lamb mince

1 onion, peeled and finely chopped

1 celery stick, trimmed and thinly sliced

1 carrot, trimmed and cut into roughly 1cm chunks

100g mushrooms, sliced

100g dried green lentils

500ml lamb or vegetable stock (fresh or made with 1 stock cube)

2 tbsp tomato purée

1 bay leaf

½ tsp dried thyme

For the topping:

300g parsnips, trimmed, washed well and cut into roughly 2cm
   chunks

1 × 400g can cannellini beans, drained and rinsed

4 tbsp full-fat crème fraîche

2–3 tbsp full-fat milk

1. Preheat the oven to 180°C/fan 160°C/gas 4.

2. Heat the oil in a flame-proof casserole (it will need to hold around 3 litres) and gently fry the lamb, onion, celery, carrot and mushrooms for 10 minutes, or until lightly browned, stirring regularly to break up the mince.

3. Add the lentils, stock, tomato purée, bay leaf and thyme and bring to a simmer. Cover with a lid, transfer to the oven and cook for 1 hour, or until the lentils are tender and the sauce is thick.

4. Meanwhile, place the parsnips in a large saucepan and cover with cold water. Bring to the boil and cook for 15–20 minutes, or until tender. Add the beans and simmer for a further 2 minutes.

5. Drain the parsnips and beans and return them to the pan. Add the crème fraîche and milk, season with flaked sea salt and plenty of freshly ground black pepper and mash together well.

6. Remove the lamb from the oven and stir well. Spoon the parsnip mixture on top, return to the oven uncovered and cook for 15 minutes, or until the parsnip mash is hot.

Cook's tip: You could transfer the cooked mince to a warmed flame-proof pie dish before topping and grilling.

Smokey fish gratin

A simple, creamy fish pie with lots of flavour and a crispy topping – comfort food rich in omega-3.

Serves 2 – 570 calories

1 tsp olive oil, for greasing

260g mixed fish pieces (including salmon, cod and smoked haddock), cut into chunks

75g frozen peas

125g full-fat crème fraîche

25g wholegrain sourdough breadcrumbs

50g Cheddar, coarsely grated

small handful chopped parsley (optional)

1. Preheat the oven to 200°C/fan 180°C/gas 6. Grease a shallow ovenproof dish with the oil. (The dish will need to be large enough to hold around 500ml.)

2. Place the fish and peas in the dish, season with a little freshly ground black pepper and toss lightly. Cover with foil and bake for 10 minutes.

3. Remove from the oven and gently stir in the crème fraîche. Mix the breadcrumbs and cheese together in a bowl, then sprinkle over the top of the fish with the parsley, if using. Return to the oven for a further 10–15 minutes, or until the crumbs are golden and the filling is bubbling.

Cook's tip: If you can't get hold of a wholegrain sourdough loaf, use any wholegrain loaf or sourdough bread to make the crumbs.

Turkey and lentil Bolognese

Enjoy this gut-friendly Bolognese with freshly cooked courgetti, or small portions of wholewheat spaghetti and lots of grated Parmesan.

Serves 4 – 415 calories

4 tbsp olive oil

1 large onion, peeled and finely chopped

150g chestnut mushrooms, sliced

300g turkey mince

2 garlic cloves, peeled and crushed

100g dried red split lentils

2 × 400g cans chopped tomatoes

150ml red wine

1 chicken stock cube

1½ tsp dried oregano

1–2 bay leaves (optional)

1. Heat the oil in a large non-stick saucepan and gently fry the onion, mushrooms and turkey mince for 5–7 minutes, or until the onion is softened and the turkey is lightly coloured, stirring regularly. Add the garlic and cook for a few seconds more, stirring.
2. Tip the lentils into the pan. Add the tomatoes, red wine, stock cube, oregano and bay leaves, if using. Pour in 200ml water and bring to a simmer. Reduce the heat and simmer gently for 30 minutes, or until the lentils are softened, the turkey is tender and the sauce is thick, stirring occasionally. Add a little extra water, if

needed. Season to taste with flaked sea salt and freshly ground black pepper to serve.

Cook's tip: There are plenty of gluten-free, high-fibre pasta alternatives, including those made using buckwheat, pea or lentil flour.

Nori-flavoured warm salmon and butternut pumpkin salad

A delicious and colourful poke bowl, with an Asian flavour and lots of texture. Full of anti-inflammatory omega-3 from the oily fish and an extra boost from the seaweed, combined with gut-friendly fibre – all of which should enhance sleep.

Serves 2 – 590 calories

300g butternut pumpkin, peeled and cut into roughly 2cm chunks

1 tbsp extra-virgin olive oil

2 salmon fillets (roughly 120g each)

100g frozen podded edamame soya beans or peas

2 large handfuls young spinach leaves (around 75g)

4 radishes, sliced, or 1 carrot, trimmed and coarsely grated

2 spring onions, trimmed and finely sliced

2 tbsp dark soy sauce

2 tsp sesame oil

For the nori seasoning:

1 nori sheet, cut into wide strips

½ tsp crushed dried chilli flakes

2 tbsp sesame seeds

good pinch ground ginger (optional)

1. Preheat oven to 200°C/fan 180°C/gas 6. Line a baking tray with non-stick baking paper.

2. Toss the pumpkin with the oil, then scatter over the prepared tray. Bake for 20 minutes.

3. Remove from the oven, turn the pumpkin and add the salmon to the tray, skin-side down. Season with freshly ground black pepper and bake for 10–12 minutes, or until the salmon is just cooked and the pumpkin is tender.

4. Meanwhile, place the nori, chilli, sesame, ginger, if using, and a good pinch of flaked sea salt in a blender and blitz into tiny pieces, without allowing it to become a powder.

5. Cook the edamame beans or peas in a pan of boiling water for 2 minutes.

6. Divide the spinach leaves, beans or peas, radishes or grated carrot and spring onions between two wide bowls. Top with the cooked pumpkin and salmon (you should be able to lift the salmon off its skin once cooked).

7. Mix the soy sauce and sesame oil in a small bowl, then drizzle over the salad. Sprinkle with a little of the nori seasoning to serve.

Cook's tip: Keep the rest of the seasoning in a sealed jar and use for other salads or to sprinkle on soups, stews and stir-fries.

For a vegetarian alternative, omit the salmon and cook an extra 100g butternut pumpkin. Top each salad with toasted flaked almonds or hazelnuts for added protein.

Veg sides

Go to sleep on your vegetables. The greener, more colourful and diverse the better. Veg, along with beans, lentils and wholegrains, are a key part of the Med-style diet – both for their taste and the huge variety of beneficial nutrients, vitamins and protein they deliver. Aim to eat 30 different varieties of vegetables, fruit and legumes a week – this is easier than you think, although build up to it gradually, as your gut may not be ready for a sudden switch.

Baked turmeric-spiced fennel and onion

Combining soluble fibre and the anti-inflammatory effects of turmeric, this juicy, delicately flavoured dish goes with almost anything.

Serves 2 – 160 calories

2 tbsp olive oil

1 tsp ground turmeric

1½ tbsp fresh lemon juice

2 small fennel bulbs (each around 225g), trimmed and sliced
   lengthways into 8

1 small onion, peeled and quartered

freshly chopped coriander, to serve (optional)

1. Preheat the oven to 200°C/fan 180°C/gas 6.
2. Place the oil, turmeric and lemon juice in a large bowl. Add a good pinch of flaked sea salt and whisk together lightly.
3. Add the fennel and onion to the bowl and toss together well. Season with freshly ground black pepper and scatter over a large baking tray in a single layer. Bake for about 25 minutes, or until the fennel is softened and lightly browned.
4. Scatter with the coriander, if using, to serve.

Braised red cabbage with walnuts and apple

Wonderful winter food. Serve with cold cooked meats or crumble microbe-rich blue cheese on top.

Serves 4 – 215 calories

1 small red cabbage (around 525g), quartered, cored and thinly
   sliced

2 tbsp extra-virgin olive oil

½ tsp flaked sea salt

2 star anise (optional)

1 cinnamon stick or 1 tsp ground cinnamon

1 cooking apple (around 200g), unpeeled, quartered, cored and cut
    into roughly 1.5cm chunks
50g soft pitted dates, thinly sliced
50g walnut halves, very roughly chopped
1½ tbsp red wine vinegar or cider vinegar

1. Place the cabbage in a large saucepan with 150ml cold water. Stir in the oil, salt and spices. Bring to a gentle simmer and cook over a low heat, covered, for 15 minutes, stirring occasionally.
2. Add the apple, dates, walnuts and vinegar and return to a simmer. Cook over a medium-high heat, uncovered, for 5 minutes, or until the liquid has almost all evaporated, stirring frequently.
3. Adjust the seasoning, adding a little more vinegar if needed. Remove the star anise and cinnamon stick to serve.

Roasted vegetables with thyme

These baked Mediterranean vegetables will help get you closer to that ideal of 30 different vegetables a week. Serve warm or cold – they are great for a packed lunch the next day, tossed with leaves or wholewheat couscous or pasta, and perhaps some halloumi or feta, and nuts and seeds.

Serves 4 – 250 calories

2 capsicums (any colour), deseeded and cut into roughly 2cm chunks
1 sweet potato (around 300g), scrubbed well and cut into roughly
    2cm chunks

2 zucchinis, trimmed and cut into roughly 2cm chunks

1 red onion, peeled and cut into 10 thin wedges

4 tbsp extra-virgin olive oil, plus extra for drizzling

1 tbsp fresh thyme leaves (roughly 2–3 sprigs)

½ tsp crushed dried chilli flakes (optional)

1. Preheat the oven to 220°C/fan 200°C/gas 7.
2. Place all the vegetables in a large bowl and toss with the oil. Season with a large pinch of flaked sea salt and lots of freshly ground black pepper. Scatter over a large baking tray in a single layer and roast for 25 minutes, or until softened and lightly browned.
3. Remove from the oven, scatter with the thyme and chilli flakes, if using, and turn all the vegetables to coat. Return to the oven for a further 5 minutes.

Seeded rainbow salad

Bitter leaves can help digestion, particularly when eaten at the start of a meal. Here you also get a wide range of anti-inflammatory phytonutrients from the different-coloured vegetables.

Serves 4 – 290 calories

100g mixed salad leaves, watercress or rocket

2 heads chicory (white or red), trimmed and very thinly sliced

100g cherry tomatoes, halved

1 capsicum (yellow or orange), deseeded and thinly sliced

2 cooked beetroot (not pickled), cut into roughly 2cm chunks

2 tbsp mixed seeds (ideally toasted – see page 232)

For the nutty dressing:

25g hazelnuts, finely chopped

10g fresh parsley, leaves finely chopped

2 tbsp cider vinegar

6 tbsp extra-virgin olive oil

1. Place the salad leaves, chicory, tomatoes and capsicum in a large serving bowl and toss lightly. Scatter with the beetroot and seeds.
2. To make the dressing, place the nuts, parsley, vinegar and oil in small bowl. Add a pinch of flaked sea salt and lots of freshly ground black pepper and whisk together. Drizzle over the salad to serve.

Smashed chickpeas

This makes a filling and tasty side dish containing lots of lovely sleep-enhancing fibre. Serve with grilled or roasted meats or fish, roasted Mediterranean vegetables or griddled eggplant.

Serves 2 – 350 calories

3 tbsp extra-virgin olive oil

1 onion, peeled and finely chopped

1 garlic clove, peeled and crushed

1 × 400g can organic chickpeas

1 tsp finely chopped fresh rosemary

100ml white wine or water (roughly 1 small glass)

1. Heat the oil in a saucepan, add the onion and gently fry for 5 minutes, or until softened, stirring regularly. Add the garlic and cook for a few seconds more.

2. Tip the chickpeas and their water into the pan, add the rosemary and wine or water and bring to a simmer. Cook for 5 minutes, stirring regularly.

3. Remove from the heat and use a stick blender to blitz until smooth. Season with flaked sea salt and freshly ground black pepper to taste, and drizzle with some extra-virgin olive oil to serve, if you like.

Spinach in garlic yoghurt

Smooth, softened spinach stirred with creamy, full-fat yoghurt. A great accompaniment to many dishes – fish, vegetable, meat or curry.

Serves 2 – 220 calories

2 tbsp extra-virgin olive oil

1 small garlic clove, peeled and crushed

100g young spinach leaves

150g full-fat live Greek yoghurt or plant-based yoghurt

2 tbsp full-fat milk or plant-based milk

large pinch sumac or toasted cumin seeds (see tip)

1. Heat 1½ tablespoons of the oil in a large saucepan, add the garlic and gently fry for 20–30 seconds, or until softened but not browned, stirring constantly.
2. Add the spinach and cook for about 2 minutes, stirring, until well softened. Tip into a serving bowl and leave to cool for at least 15 minutes.
3. Add the yoghurt and milk to the cold spinach, season with a good pinch of flaked sea salt and plenty of freshly ground black pepper. Stir together well.
4. Drizzle with the remaining oil and sprinkle with sumac or toasted cumin seeds to serve.

Cook's tip: Toast the cumin seeds in a dry frying pan over a medium heat for 1–2 minutes, stirring constantly, to enhance the flavour.

Treats

Move away from sweetened, sugary, processed foods and snacks as much as you can. They are damaging for your delicate microbiome and, even if you eat healthily most of the time, you can undo the benefits quite quickly by eating the bad stuff.

The 'treats' here have no added sugar; instead, they use whole fruits and the occasional dash of honey or maple syrup to add sweetness.

Fruit is a great source of vitamins and fibre and contains a huge variety of chemicals with antioxidant and anti-inflammatory properties, which are particularly concentrated in and around the skin, so eat as much of the fruit as you can.

Aim to eat a couple of portions of fruit a day – ideally after a meal when they are less likely to spike your blood sugars. Lower-sugar varieties, such as berries and apples and pears, are best. But, as with veg, variety is good.

Dorset apple cake

A delicious, tangy cake, adapted from the classic Dorset apple cake recipe to give it a gut-friendly twist.

Serves 12 – 265 calories

2 small–medium eating apples

1 tbsp fresh lemon juice

1 tsp ground cinnamon

3 large eggs

150g butter, softened

200g ground almonds

50g self-raising brown flour

100g large soft pitted dates, finely chopped

1 tsp vanilla extract

1 tsp baking powder

20g flaked almonds

1. Preheat the oven to 190°C/fan 170°C/gas 5. Grease and line a 23cm round loose-based cake tin with baking parchment.

2. Core the apples and cut each one into about 12 wedges (keeping the skin on). Place in a medium bowl and toss with the lemon juice and cinnamon.

3. Place the eggs, butter, ground almonds, flour, half the dates, vanilla extract and baking powder in a food processor and blitz until smooth. Remove the blade and stir in the rest of the dates.

4. Spoon the batter into the prepared tin and spread to the sides.

Top with the apple wedges, tucking them fairly close to each other in concentric circles, and bake for 25 minutes.

5. Remove from the oven, sprinkle with the flaked almonds and cook for a further 12–15 minutes, or until the cake is cooked through, the apples are tender and the nuts are golden.

6. Cool in the tin for 30 minutes before removing. Cut into slender slices to serve.

Banana on toast with crunchy walnuts

If you need an instant filler after a meal, this is easy, healthy comfort food.

Serves 1 – 325 calories

1 handful walnut halves (around 20g), roughly chopped

1 thin slice seeded sourdough

20g full-fat soft cheese (around 1 tbsp), such as Philadelphia

1 small banana, peeled and sliced

pinch ground cinnamon (optional)

1. Place the walnuts in a dry frying pan over a medium heat. Toast for 2–3 minutes, or until hot and lightly browned, stirring regularly.

2. Meanwhile, toast the sourdough and spread with the soft cheese.

3. Top with the sliced banana and scatter with the toasted walnuts. Sprinkle with a little ground cinnamon, if you like, to serve.

Zucchini, orange and apricot cake

Zinging with orange flavour and remarkably low in sugar, this cake is scrumptious and microbiome-friendly. Serve in small squares like a brownie.

Makes 20 servings – 145 calories

100g coconut oil, melted, plus extra for greasing

4 medium eggs

150g ready-to-eat dried apricots, roughly chopped

2 tsp vanilla extract

2 small zucchinis (roughly 250g total weight), trimmed and
  coarsely grated

100g self-raising brown flour

150g ground almonds

1 tsp mixed spice

1½ tsp baking powder

finely grated zest 1 large orange

3 balls stem ginger in syrup, drained and finely chopped

1. Preheat the oven to 180°C/fan 160°C/gas 4. Lightly oil and line the base of a 23cm loose-based square cake tin with non-stick baking paper.

2. Place the eggs, apricots, melted coconut oil and vanilla extract in a large bowl and blitz with a stick blender (or blend in a food processor), until the apricots are very finely chopped and the eggs are pale. Add half the grated zucchini, the flour, ground almonds, mixed spice and baking powder and blitz again.

3. Stir in the orange zest, remaining zucchini and the ginger.

4. Spoon into the tin and spread to the sides. Bake for 30–35 minutes, or until risen, golden brown and firm to the touch.

5. Cool in the tin for 10 minutes, then turn out and leave to cool on a wire rack. Cut into small squares to serve.

Cook's tip: This cake keeps well for 2–3 days wrapped in foil. Extra squares can be frozen.

Nutty berry crunch

Healthy berries, nuts and wholegrain fibre. Serve with full-fat crème fraîche or live Greek yoghurt.

Serves 5 – 230 calories

500g frozen summer berries or mixed fresh berries

50g ready-to-eat dried apricots, finely chopped

1 tbsp honey

For the topping:

40g butter or coconut oil

40g plain wholemeal flour

40g jumbo porridge oats

40g flaked almonds

½ tsp ground cinnamon

1. Preheat the oven to 200°C/fan 180°C/gas 6.
2. Place the frozen berries in a shallow 1-litre pie dish. Add 4–5 tablespoons water, the apricots and honey and toss together.
3. To make the topping, rub together the butter or coconut oil, flour, oats, almonds, cinnamon and a pinch of salt in a large bowl until well combined. Sprinkle this mixture over the fruit.
4. Place the pie dish on a baking tray and bake for 30–40 minutes, or until the filling is hot and the topping is lightly browned.

Cook's tip: Try and ensure your berries include strawberries for their natural sweetness.

Fermented vegetables

Fun, cheap and easy to make, home-fermented foods are becoming increasingly popular, valued for their sweet, tangy flavours as well as their rich probiotic qualities.

Fermenting your own veg gives you variety, flavour and far more healthy bugs than almost anything you will find in a supermarket. Experiment with your own variations of different vegetables and spices.

Fill the fridge with jars of colourful veg. You may produce more wind as your microbiome adjusts, so eat smaller quantities at first. And use them with caution or avoid them altogether if you have reduced immunity.

The jar(s) need to be clean but not sterilised and the same goes for your hands. The salt kills most bacteria, other than the acid- and salt-loving bacteria you need for fermenting. Ideally use organic veg.

No calorie counts here – ferments can be considered 'free' foods ...

Purple pickled onions

This is one of our favourites – juicy, sweet and salty pink onion rings bring crunch and flavour to almost any savoury meal. Technically, they are fermented rather than pickled in vinegar – which means they taste better, as well as enhancing your microbiome.

¼ small beetroot, peeled

2 large organic red onions, peeled and thinly sliced into rings

3 tsp flaked sea salt, such as Maldon

1 × 500ml jar with a well-fitting lid, cleaned

pinch coriander seeds

½ tsp peppercorns

1. Grate the beetroot onto a board, then put in a bowl. Add the onions and salt in a few layers.
2. Using your hands (you may need gloves to avoid staining), massage the salt into the onions and beetroot. Leave for 30 minutes to two hours for the juices to appear.
3. Stuff the onion mixture firmly into the jar, sprinkling coriander seeds and peppercorns between the layers as you go, until it's full, adding any remaining fluid. Using a blunt object, like the end of a rolling pin or the back of a spoon, press down on the vegetables to release air bubbles and submerge them in the fluid. If not enough fluid is produced to cover the veg, add 1 tablespoon at a time of filtered (non-chlorinated) water to top it up until it reaches 1.5–2cm below the top of the jar.

4. Close the lid firmly and keep the onions at room temperature for 5–10 days. Release the gasses 1–2 times a day, particularly in the first few days, pressing down to release more bubbles. (This is called 'burping'.) Refrigerate to slow the fermentation and they should last for 2–3 months. Remove anything that becomes mouldy or blackened and throw it away if it smells bad. It should have a slightly sweet yeasty and tart smell.

Fennel and onion

A great way to get two of the best prebiotic vegetables, with all their biome-friendly properties.

  2 good-sized fennel bulbs, finely sliced

  2 small-medium onions, finely sliced

  2 tsp flaked sea salt, such as Maldon

  1 × 500ml jar with a well-fitting lid, cleaned

  1 tsp black peppercorns

  ½–1 tsp crushed dried chilli flakes

1. Place the fennel and onions in a large bowl, and massage the salt in with your hands. Leave for 30 minutes to two hours for the juices to appear.

2. Stuff the veg mixture into the jar, adding any remaining fluid. Using a blunt object, like the end of a rolling pin or the back of a spoon, press down on the veg to release air bubbles and submerge

them. If there is not enough fluid to cover the veg, make up 200ml of filtered or spring water with 1 teaspoon salt and add this 1 tablespoon at a time until it reaches 1.5–2cm below the top of the jar.

3. Add the peppercorns and chilli and close the lid firmly. Keep at room temperature for 5–10 days. Release the gases 1–2 times a day, particularly in the first few days, pressing down to release more bubbles. Refrigerate to slow the fermentation and they should last for 2–3 months. Remove anything that becomes mouldy or blackened and throw it away if it smells bad. It should have a slightly sweet yeasty and tart smell.

Endnotes

1   NREM sleep as a novel protective cognitive reserve factor in the face of Alzheimer's disease pathology. BMC Medicine, 2023; 21 (1) DOI: 10.1186/s12916-023-02811-

2   Prefrontal atrophy, disrupted NREM slow waves and impaired hippocampal-dependent memory in aging. *Nature Neuroscience*, 2013. https://www.ncbi.nlm.nih.gov/pubmed/23354332

3   The effects of partial sleep deprivation on energy balance. *Eur J Clin Nutr*, 2016. https://www.ncbi.nlm.nih.gov/pubmed/27804960

4   Acute sleep restriction increases dietary intake in preschool-age children. *J of Sleep Research*, 2015. https://onlinelibrary.wiley.com/doi/full/10.1111/jsr.12450

5   Associations between short sleep duration and central obesity in women. *Sleep*, 2010. https://www.ncbi.nlm.nih.gov/pubmed/20469801

6   The impact of sleep on female sexual response and behavior. *J of Sexual Medicine*, 2015. https://onlinelibrary.wiley.com/doi/full/10.1111/jsm.12858

7   Sex and sleep: perceptions of sex as a sleep promoting behavior in the general adult population. *Frontiers in Public Health*, 2019. https://www.frontiersin.org/articles/10.3389/fpubh.2019.00033/full

8   Validity, potential clinical utility and comparison of a consumer activity tracker and a research-grade activity tracker in insomnia disorder II: Outside the laboratory. *J of Sleep Research*, 2020. https://www.ncbi.nlm.nih.gov/pubmed/31680327

9   Gender and time for sleep among U.S. adults. *Am Sociol Rev*, 2013. https://www.ncbi.nlm.nih.gov/pmc/articles/PMC4164903

10 A marker for the end of adolescence. *Current Biology*, Vol 14. https://www.cell.com/current-biology/pdf/S0960-9822(04)00928-5.pdf

11 School start time change, sleep duration and driving accidents in highschool students. *Chest J*, 2019 https://journal.chestnet.org/article/S0012-3692(19)30482-9/fulltext

12 Resetting the late timing of 'night owls' has a positive impact on mental health and performance. Sleep Medicine, 2019. https://www.sciencedirect.com/science/article/abs/pii/S1389945719301388

13 Entrainment of the human circadian clock to the natural light-dark cycle. *Current Biology*, 2013. https://www.ncbi.nlm.nih.gov/pubmed/23910656

14 In short photoperiods, human sleep is biphasic. *J of Sleep Research*, 1992. https://www.ncbi.nlm.nih.gov/pubmed/10607034

15 Truck drivers should be routinely tested for sleep apnoea. *Guardian*, 2019. https://www.theguardian.com/society/2019/sep/30/truck-drivers-should-be-routinely-tested-for-sleep-apnoea

16 Lifestyle intervention with weight reduction; First-line treatment in mild obstructive sleep apnea. *AJRCCM*, 2019. https://www.atsjournals.org/doi/full/10.1164/rccm.200805-669OC

17 Experimental 'jet lag' inhibits adult neurogenesis and produces long-term cognitive deficits in female hamsters. *PLoS One*, 2010. https://journals.plos.org/plosone/article?id=10.1371/journal.pone.0015267

18 Melatonin for the prevention and treatment of jet lag. *Cochrane*, 2002. https://www.cochranelibrary.com/cdsr/doi/10.1002/14651858.CD001520/full

19 Using the Argonne diet in jet lag prevention. *Military Medicine*, 2002. https://www.ncbi.nlm.nih.gov/pubmed/12099077

20 Common sleep disorders increase risk of motor vehicle crashes and adverse health outcomes in firefighters. *J of Clinical Sleep Medicine*, 2015. http://jcsm.aasm.org/ViewAbstract.aspx?pid=29921

21 Sleep disorders, health, and safety in police officers. *JAMA*, 2011. https://jamanetwork.com/journals/jama/fullarticle/1104746

22 Optimal shift duration and sequence. *American J of Public Health*, 2007. https://www.ncbi.nlm.nih.gov/pmc/articles/PMC1854972

23 Workplace interventions to promote sleep health and an alert, healthy workforce. *J of Clinical Sleep Medicine*, 2019. https://www.ncbi.nlm.nih.gov/pmc/articles/PMC6457507

24 The impact of sleep timing and bright light exposure on attentional impairment during night work. *J of Biological Rhythms*, 2008. https://pubmed.ncbi.nlm.nih.gov/18663241-the-impact-of-sleep-timing-and-bright-light-exposure-on-attentional-impairment-during-night-work

25 Does modifying the timing of meal intake improve cardiovascular risk factors? *BMJ Open*. https://bmjopen.bmj.com/content/8/3/e020396

26 Shift work, role overload, and the transition to parenthood. *Wiley Online*, 2007. https://onlinelibrary.wiley.com/doi/full/10.1111/j.1741-3737.2006.00349.x

27 Modafinil for excessive sleepiness associated with chronic shift work sleep disorder. *Prim Care Companion J Clin Psych*, 2007. https://www.ncbi.nlm.nih.gov/pmc/articles/PMC1911168

28 Modafinil increases the latency of response in the Hayling Sentence Completion Test in healthy volunteers. *PLoS One*. https://journals.plos.org/plosone/article?id=10.1371/journal.pone.0110639

29 Why lack of sleep is bad for your health. *NHS*, 2018. https://www.nhs.uk/live-well/sleep-and-tiredness/why-lack-of-sleep-is-bad-for-your-health/

30 Sleep patterns and school performance of Korean adolescents assessed using a Korean version of the pediatric daytime sleepiness scale. *Korean J of Pediatrics*, 2011. https://www.ncbi.nlm.nih.gov/pmc/articles/PMC3040363

31 In US, 40% get less than recommended amount of sleep. *Wellbeing*, 2013. https://news.gallup.com/poll/166553/less-recommended-amount-sleep.aspx

32 Sleep health of Australian adults in 2016: results of the 2016 Sleep Health Foundation national survey. *Sleep Health*, 2017. https://pubmed.ncbi.nlm.nih.gov/28346149/

33 Associations of longitudinal sleep trajectories with risky sexual behavior during late sdolescence. *Health Psychol*, 2019. https://www.ncbi.nlm.nih.gov/pubmed/31157533

34 Long-term effects of pregnancy and childbirth on sleep satisfaction and duration of first-time and experienced mothers and fathers. *Sleep*, 2019. https://www.ncbi.nlm.nih.gov/pubmed/30649536

35 Menopause and sleep. *Sleep Foundation*. https://www.sleepfoundation.org/articles/menopause-and-sleep

36 Benefits and safety of dietary protein for bone health – an expert consensus paper endorsed by the European Society for Clinical and Economical Aspects of Osteoporosis, Osteoarthritis, and Musculoskeletal Diseases and by the International Osteoporosis Foundation. *Osteoporosis Int.*, 2018. https://pubmed.ncbi.nlm.nih.gov/29740667/

37 Health related quality of life after combined hormone replacement therapy. *BMJ*, 2008. https://www.bmj.com/content/337/bmj.a1190.abstract

38 Physiological correlates of prolonged sleep deprivation in rats. *Science*, 1983. https://science.sciencemag.org/content/221/4606/182

39 The boy who stayed awake for 11 days. *BBC*, 2018. https://www.bbc.com/future/article/20180118-the-boy-who-stayed-awake-for-11-days

40 Night watch in one brain hemisphere during sleep associated with the first-night effect in humans. *Current Biology*, 2016. https://www.cell.com/current-biology/fulltext/ S0960-9822(16)30174-9#%20

41 A rare mutation of B1-Adrenergic Receptor affects sleep/wake behaviors. *Neuron*, 2019. https://www.cell.com/neuron/fulltext/S0896-6273(19)30652-X

42 The dangers of doctors driving home. *Guardian*, 2016. https://www.theguardian.com/ healthcare-network/2016/jul/26/two-in-five-doctors-fallen-asleep-wheel-night-shift

43 Acute sleep deprivation and culpable motor vehicle crash involvement. *Sleep*, 2018. https://www.ncbi.nlm.nih.gov/pubmed/30239905

44 Daylight savings time and myocardial infarction. *BMJ*, 2014 https://openheart.bmj.com/content/1/1/e000019

45 Spring forward at your own risk: Daylight saving time and fatal vehicle crashes. *American Economic J*, 2016. https://pubs.aeaweb.org/doi/pdfplus/10.1257/app.20140100

46 Sleepy punishers are harsh punishers: Daylight saving time and legal sentences. *APA PsycNet*, 2017. https://psycnet.apa.org/record/2017-06044-010

47 Effects of initiating moderate alcohol intake on cardiometabolic risk in adults with type 2 diabetes. *Ann Intern Med*, 2015. https://www.ncbi.nlm.nih.gov/pubmed/26458258

48 Beneficial effects of low alcohol exposure, but adverse effects of high alcohol intake on glymphatic function. *Open Access*, 2018. https://www.nature.com/articles/s41598-018-20424-y

49 Before-bedtime passive body heating by warm shower or bath to improve sleep. *Sleep Medicine Reviews*, 2019. https://www.sciencedirect.com/science/article/abs/ pii/S1087079218301552?via%3Dihub

50 Can music help you calm down and sleep better? *Sleep Foundation*. https://www.sleepfoundation.org/articles/can-music-help-you-calm-down-and-sleep-better

51 The effects of bedtime writing on difficulty falling asleep: A polysomnographic study comparing to-do lists and completed activity lists. *J Exp Psychol Gen*, 2018. https://www.ncbi.nlm.nih.gov/pmc/articles/PMC5758411/

52 Insomnia: Pharmacologic therapy. *Am Fam Physician*, 2017. https://www.ncbi.nlm. nih. gov/pubmed/28671376

53 Australian public assessment report for melatonin. 2011. https://www. tga.gov.au/ sites/default/files/auspar-circadin-110118.pdf

54 Circadin 2 mg prolonged-release tablets. https://www.medicines.org.uk/emc/ product/2809/smpc

55 A systematic review of the effect of inhaled essential oils on sleep. *J Alt and Comp Medicine*, 2014. https://www.liebertpub.com/doi/10.1089/acm.2013.0311

56 Runner-up: Tim Cook, the technologist. *Time*, 2012. https://poy.time.com/2012/ 12/19/runner-up-tim-cook-the-technologist/2

57 This is when successful people wake up. *HuffPost*. https://www.huffpost.com/entry/ this-is-when-successful-people-wake-up_b_596d17a3e4b0376db8b65a1a

58 The effect of resistance exercise on sleep. *Sleep Medicine Reviews*, 2018. https://www. sciencedirect.com/science/article/abs/pii/S1087079216301526

59 Effect of breakfast on weight and energy intake: Systematic review and meta-analysis of randomised controlled trials. *BMJ*, 2019. https://www.bmj.com/content/364/ bmj.l42

60 Fiber and saturated fat are associated with sleep arousals and slow wave sleep. *J of Clinical Sleep Medicine*, 2016. https://jcsm.aasm.org/ViewAbstract.aspx?pid=30412

61 Effects of diet on sleep quality. *Advances in Nutrition*, 2016. https://www.ncbi.nlm. nih.gov/pmc/articles/PMC5015038

62 A randomised controlled trial of dietary improvement for adults with major depression (the 'SMILES' trial). *BMC Medicine*, 2017. https://bmcmedicine. biomedcentral.com/ articles/10.1186/s12916-017-0791-y

63 Gut microbiome diversity is associated with sleep physiology in humans. *PLoS One*, 2019. https://www.ncbi.nlm.nih.gov/pubmed/31589627

64 Effects of a tart cherry juice beverage on the sleep of older adults with insomnia. *J of Medicinal Food*, 2010. https://www.liebertpub.com/doi/abs/10.1089/ jmf.2009.0096

65 Effect of kiwifruit consumption on sleep quality in adults with sleep problems. *Asia Pacific J of Clinical Nutrition*, 2011. https://www.ncbi.nlm.nih.gov/ pubmed/21669584

66 Sweet dreams are made of cheese. *Scitable*, 2013. https://www.nature.com/scitable/ blog/mind-read/sweet_dreams_are_made_of

67 Primary prevention of cardiovascular disease with a Mediterranean diet. *New England J of Medicine*, 2013. https://www.nejm.org/doi/full/10.1056/NEJMoa1200303

68 Adherence to the Mediterranean diet is associated with better sleep quality in Italian adults. *Nutrients*, 2019. https://www.ncbi.nlm.nih.gov/pmc/articles/PMC6566275/

69 Mediterranean healthy eating, aging, and lifestyles (MEAL) study. *International J of Food Sciences and Nutrition*, 2017. https://www.ncbi.nlm.nih.gov/pubmed/27919168

70 Mediterranean diet pattern and sleep duration and insomnia symptoms in the Multi-Ethnic Study of Atherosclerosis. *Sleep*, 2018. https://www.ncbi.nlm.nih.gov/pmc/articles/PMC6231522/

71 Fiber and saturated fat are associated with sleep arousals and slow wave sleep. *Journal of Clinical Sleep Medicine*, 2016. https://jcsm.aasm.org/ViewAbstract.aspx?pid=30412

72 A randomised controlled trial of dietary improvement for adults with major depression (the 'SMILES' trial). *BMC Medicine*, 2017. https://bmcmedicine.biomedcentral.com/articles/10.1186/s12916-017-0791-y

73 Red meat consumption and mood anxiety disorders. *APA PsycNet*, 2012. https://psycnet.apa.org/record/2012-15003-012

74 A Mediterranean-style dietary intervention supplemented with fish oil improves diet quality and mental health in people with depression (HELFIMED). *Nutritional Neuroscience*, 2019. https://www.ncbi.nlm.nih.gov/pubmed/29215971

75 Scientists bust myth that our bodies have more bacteria than human cells. *Nature*, 2016. https://www.nature.com/news/scientists-bust-myth-that-our-bodies-have-more-bacteria-than-human-cells-1.19136

76 Gut microbiome diversity is associated with sleep physiology in humans. *PLoS One*, 2019. https://www.ncbi.nlm.nih.gov/pubmed/31589627

77 Enhancing influence of intranasal interleukin-6 on slow-wave activity and memory consolidation during sleep. *Faseb J*, 2009. https://www.fasebj.org/doi/10.1096/fj.08-122853

78 Association between maternal fermented food consumption and infant sleep duration. *PLoS One*, 2019. https://www.ncbi.nlm.nih.gov/pubmed/31584958

79 Effects of probiotics on cognitive reactivity, mood, and sleep quality. *Front Psychiatry*, 2019. https://www.ncbi.nlm.nih.gov/pmc/articles/PMC6445894

80 Ten-hour time-restricted eating reduces weight, blood pressure, and atherogenic lipids in patients with metabolic syndrome. *ScienceDirect*, 2010. https://www. sciencedirect.com/ science/article/pii/S1550413119306114

81 Treatment of chronic insomnia by restriction of time in bed. *Sleep*, 1987. https:// www.ncbi.nlm.nih.gov/pubmed/3563247

82 The evidence base of sleep restriction therapy for treating insomnia disorder. *Sleep Medicine Reviews*, 2014. https://www.ncbi.nlm.nih.gov/pubmed/24629826

83 Meta-analysis of the antidepressant effects of acute sleep deprivation. *J of Clinical Psychiatry*, 2017. https://www.ncbi.nlm.nih.gov/pubmed/28937707

Index

4-Week Sleep Plan: summary 12–13, 218–20
5:2 diet 34, 63–4
16:8 diet 118
20-minute getting up 129, 130, 133

abdominal fat 36, 176, 220, 223
accidents: car crashes 53–4, 83, 102, 106–7
  sleepwalking 66–9
acid reflux 119
adenosine 45, 103, 115
ADRB1 gene 105
adrenaline 30
aerobic exercise 217
ageing: amount of deep sleep 25, 29
  memory 28–9
  microbiome and 94, 155
  shift work 81, 84
  sleep deprivation 93–4
  snoring 61, 93
aggression 92
alcohol 120–1, 193–4, 196
almonds: black grapes with yoghurt and almonds 224–5
  nutty berry crunch 287–8
  rosy overnight oats 226
alternate-nostril breathing 207–8
Alzheimer's disease 25–6, 63

amitriptyline 127
amygdalae 30
anchovies: cheesy celeriac and anchovy bake 261–2
  hot-smoked salmon, anchovies, artichoke and broccoli pasta 244–5
anti-snoring devices 66
antihistamines 127–8
antioxidants 152
anxiety 40, 126–7, 135, 149, 150–1, 206–9
apnoea, sleep 36, 61–5, 79
appetite and hormones 34–5, 176
apples 160
  braised red cabbage with walnuts and apple 277–8
  Dorset apple cake 284–5
  rosy overnight oats 226
apps 209
apricots: zucchini, orange and apricot cake 286–7
  rosy overnight oats 226
Archer, Dr Simon 50
Argonne diet 75–7
artichokes: hot-smoked salmon, anchovies, artichoke and broccoli pasta 244–5
Aserinsky, Eugene 19–20
Augean stables 24

Automatic Negative Thoughts (ANTs) 206
avocados 128
    black bean salad with lime and avocado
        252–3
    Dr Tim's hot-smoked salmon salad 239
    nori rolled crab 254–5

Bacteroidetes 142, 156
Bailey, Dr Clare: junior doctor shifts 3,
        70–1, 105
    parasomnia 3–4, 66–7
bakes: cheesy celeriac and anchovy bake
        261–2
    chicken and veg tray bake 262–3
banana on toast with crunchy walnuts 285
barley 160
baths 122–3, 128, 205
beans 158, 163
    black bean salad with lime and avocado
        252–3
    Dr Tim's hot-smoked salmon salad 239
    nori-flavoured warm salmon and
        butternut pumpkin salad 273–5
    ratatouille with white beans 267–8
    shepherd's pie with parsnip and white
        bean mash 269–70
bed: association with sleep 10, 111, 130
    invention of 98–9
    mattresses 178
bedrooms 178–9, 195
    darkness in 179
    temptation removal 115–16, 179, 182
bedtime: before midnight 26, 114
    establishing good habits 113–15
    routines 117–25, 205
    SRT and 188–90
    wind-down routine 117–21
beef 97
    beef and Jerusalem artichoke casserole
        260–1

beetroot: purple pickled onions 290–1
    seeded rainbow salad 279–80
    smoked mackerel, beetroot and tahini
        pitta 251–2
belly breathing 131
benzodiazepines 126–7
Berger, Hans 18–19
berries: nutty berry crunch 287–8
    rosy overnight oats 226
beta amyloid protein 25–6
beta-glucan 160
Bezos, Jeff 135
Bifidobacterium 155, 161, 165
Bimuno 161–3, 173
biphasic sleeping 58–60, 133
blood circulation 123
blood pressure 36, 103, 131
blood sugar levels 49, 195
    coffee and 47, 48
    measurement of 176–7, 215–16
    sleep deprivation and 33–5, 103
blue light 116, 121–2
body temperature 22, 49, 118, 123
Bolognese, turkey and lentil 272–3
brain: deep sleep and brain cleaning
        24–7
    EEG monitoring 18–20, 104
    effect of insomnia on 110
    evolutionary development 99
    glymphatic system 25, 120
    historical beliefs about sleep 17
    inflammation 148–9
    neurons 23, 32–3
    poor sleep effects 2
    rewards 35
    sleep level on each side 104
    storage capacity 27
    suprachiasmatic nucleus (SCN) 48–9,
        125
    see also memory

bread: banana on toast with crunchy
  walnuts 285
  prawns and red cabbage slaw on
    sourdough 250–1
  sardines on seeded sourdough 245
breakfast 137–8, 224–9
breathing: mindfulness 208–9
sleep apnoea 36, 62
sleep stages 23
  yogic 130–1, 185, 207–8
broccoli: Dr Tim's hot-smoked salmon
    salad 239
  hot-smoked salmon, anchovies,
    artichoke and broccoli pasta 244–5
bulgur wheat: tabbouleh with goat's
    cheese 256–7
Burnet, Prof Phil 161–3
Bush, George W. 73
butternut pumpkin: nori-flavoured warm
    salmon and butternut pumpkin salad
    273–5
butyrate 154

cabbage: braised red cabbage with walnuts
    and apple 277–8
  prawns and red cabbage slaw on
    sourdough 250–1
caffeine 45–6, 47–8, 107, 111, 183,
    193–4, 194
cakes: zucchini, orange and apricot cake
    286–7
  Dorset apple cake 284–5
camping 56
capsicums: cashew, ricotta and red
    capsicum dip 249–50
  cauliflower and roasted red capsicum
    soup 230–1
  seeded rainbow salad 279–80
car accidents 53–4, 83, 102, 106–7

cashew nuts 128, 163
  cashew, ricotta and red capsicum dip
    249–50
  oaty nutty shake 225
casserole, beef and Jerusalem artichoke
    260–1
cats 99
cauliflower and roasted red capsicum soup
    230–1
CBT (Cognitive Behavioural Therapy)
    132, 190
celeriac: cheesy celeriac and anchovy bake
    261–2
  trout with celeriac mash 258–9
celery with blue cheese dip 248–9
cerebrospinal fluid 25
cheese 164
  baked chicory with prosciutto 238
  blue cheese dip 248–9
  cheesy celeriac and anchovy bake
    261–2
  griddled eggplant with feta and pine
    nuts 241–2
  meatballs with feta and eggplant
    264–6
  nightmares myth 143–4
  pasta with peas and goat's cheese
    242–3
  smokey fish gratin 270–1
  sweet potato savoury muffins with feta
    228–9
  tabbouleh with goat's cheese 256–7
cherries 143
chicken 97
  anti-inflammatory Chinese-style
    chicken broth 233–4
  chicken and veg tray bake 262–3
  chicken noodles with pak choi 234–5
  chicken tagine with chickpeas and dates
    263–4

chickpeas 158, 163
  chicken tagine with chickpeas and dates
    263–4
  mushroom, chickpea and kale curry
    266–7
  smashed chickpeas 280–1
chicory 158
  baked chicory with prosciutto 238
  seeded rainbow salad 279–80
children: effect on parents' sleep
    92–3
  larks and owls 52–53
  parasomnia 67–8
  recommended quantity of sleep
    88
  sleep deprivation 35
  SRT 172
  synthetic melatonin 126
chlorphenamine 127–8
chocolate 161
cholesterol 36, 160
chronotypes 50, 51, 52, 81
circadian clock 185
  adjusting from owl to lark 54–6
  function of 48–9
  jet lag and 72–4
  meal times 117–19
  sleep deprivation 103
The Clever Guts Diet 112, 141, 164
clock changes 107–8
clock watching 179
cocoa 118–19, 161
coffee 46–8, 107, 111, 183
Cognitive Behavioural Therapy (CBT)
    132, 190
cognitive tests, sleep deprivation 101–4
COMISA 63
computer screens 116
contraception, effect on caffeine
    processing 46

Cook, Tim 134
cortisol 35, 37, 45, 49, 176
  CAR (cortisol arousal response) 47–8
Corynebacterium 156
CPAP machines (Continuous Positive
    Airway Pressure) 64–5
crab, nori rolled 254–5
cravings 34–5, 94, 95
creativity 31–2
criminal sentencing 108
crunches 200
curry: curried lentil soup with turmeric
    236–7
  mushroom, chickpea and kale curry
    266–7
curtains 179
cytokines 23, 157

darkness 179
dates, chicken tagine with chickpeas and
    263–4
daytime sleep 83
  see also naps
death from sleep deprivation 99, 100–1
decision making 32
deep sleep 21, 23
  and brain cleaning 24–7
  function in the body 23–4, 25
  memory function 27–9
dementia 2, 25–6, 63, 121, 149
depression 2, 37, 142, 149–50, 192
diabetes risk factors: metabolic syndrome
    36
  poor sleep effects 2
  prediabetes 176
  shift work 78
  sleep deprivation 34
diary keeping 40–1, 123–4, 172–3,
    174–5, 181, 182
Dickens, Charles 133–4, 144

diets: Argonne diet 75–7
  Mediterranean diet 144–52, 220, 223,
    276
  raw food diet 104
  time restricted eating (TRE) 117–19
  see also microbiome
dinner 139
diphenhydramine 128
dips: blue cheese dip 248–9
  cashew, ricotta and red capsicum dip
    249–50
divorce 84
dogs 99
dolphins 104
dopamine 154
Dorset apple cake 284–5
dreams: discovery of REM sleep 19–20
  emotions 29–31
drinks: alcohol 120–1, 193–4
  caffeine 45–6, 47–8, 107, 111, 183,
    193–4
  late night 118–19
drowsiness 45

eating: body temperature and 118
  meal times 49, 118, 137–8, 139, 166,
    214
edamame beans: Dr Tim's hot-smoked
    salmon salad 239
  nori-flavoured warm salmon and
    butternut pumpkin salad 273–5
  super-speedy mushroom risotto with
    edamame 246–7
Edison, Thomas 17, 87
EEG (electroencephalography) 18–20,
    104
eggplants: griddled eggplants with feta
    and pine nuts 241–2
  meatballs with feta and eggplant 264–6
  ratatouille with white beans 267–8

eggs 96–7
  scrambled with kimchi 227
Ehret, Dr Charles 75
Ekirch, Prof Roger 58, 59
employers: shift work 81
emulsifiers 155
essential oils 128–9
euphoria 103
evolution: brain alertness in sleep 104
  sleep patterns 59, 71–2
exams 28, 85
exercise 197–201
  aerobic 217
  benefits of 197
  HIIT exercises 210–11, 216, 217
  increasing activity 197, 204–5, 216
  and microbiome diversity 155
  morning routines 135, 183
  planning 198–9
  resistance 135, 185, 199–201, 204, 205
  sleep effects 197–8
  time of day 197

faeces 152, 155–6
Fast 800 65, 75, 177, 227
Fast Argonne diet 76–7
Fast Strength 199–201
fat, body: abdominal 36, 176, 220, 223
  ageing and 61
  sleep quality 35–6
Fatal Familial Insomnia (FFI) 100–1
fats, dietary 119, 148
fear response 30
fennel: baked turmeric-spiced fennel and
    onion 276–7
  fermented fennel and onion 291–2
fermented foods 164, 178, 289–92
fibre 141, 223
  fermented foods 178
  fruit 283

Mediterranean diet 2
microbiome and 153, 154, 165
prebiotics 157–63
sleep quality 14
'fight or flight' hormones 30
fish 97
    baked sweet potato with smoked
        mackerel 240
    cheesy celeriac and anchovy bake 261–2
    Dr Tim's hot-smoked salmon salad 239
    hot-smoked salmon, anchovies,
        artichoke and broccoli pasta 244–5
    nori-flavoured warm salmon and
        butternut pumpkin salad 273–5
    sardines on seeded sourdough 245
    smoked mackerel, beetroot and tahini
        pitta 251–2
    smokey fish gratin 270–1
    trout with celeriac mash 258–9
Fisher, Carrie 62
Fitbits 39–40, 42
flaxseeds 160
food: and biological clock 49
    emulsifiers 155
    fermented foods 164, 178, 289–92
    junk food 52, 63, 82, 92, 148, 155,
        195
    magnesium sources 128
    and the microbiome 203
    prebiotics 157–63
    and sleep 14, 141–67
    temptation removal 115, 116
fruit 160, 283
    see also individual types of fruit

GABA 154, 156
galactooligosaccharide (GOS) 161–3
Gardner, Randy 101–2
garlic 158
gender differences 42, 52

genes: caffeine processing 46–7
    Fatal Familial Insomnia (FFI) 100–1
    larks and 50–1
    need for little sleep 105
    testing 47
ghrelin 96, 176
glymphatic system 25, 120
grapes: black grapes with yoghurt and
        almonds 224–5
gratin, smokey fish 270–1
gratitude journal 124, 203–4
Greek mythology 24–5
growth hormone 23
gut bacteria see microbiome
gut lining repair 119, 154

hallucinations 100, 101, 104
heart disease 62, 63, 78, 83, 97
heart rate 23
Heracles 24
herbal supplements 127
herbs: tabbouleh with goat's cheese 256–7
HIIT exercises 199–201, 210–11, 216,
        217
hippocampus 27–8, 29, 73
history: attitudes to sleep 1, 17–18
    EEG monitoring 18–20
    pre-industrial sleep patterns 58–9
Hormone Replacement Therapy (HRT)
        98
hormones: appetite 34–5, 176
    circadian clock 49, 55, 56, 103
    'fight or flight' 30
    growth hormone 23
    menopause 94
    and the microbiome 112, 154, 156, 203
    REM sleep 30
    sex 37
    stress 35
    waking 45

hunger 34–5, 49, 94, 95, 176
hunter-gatherers 59, 122
hypersomnia 62
hypnagogic jerks 23
hypnograms 21
hypothalamus 48

IBS 159, 163, 165
immune system 23–4, 153, 157
infections, and sleep deprivation 24
inflammation 148–9, 152, 154, 215
insomnia: Fatal Familial Insomnia (FFI)
    100–1
  genes 46–7
  menopause 94–8
  Michael's experience 2, 4, 57–8, 59–60,
    130
  rules to follow 219–20
  test questionnaire 109–10
  types of 57, 110–11
  worrying and 129
  see also Sleep Restriction Therapy
    (SRT)
insulin 37, 118
interleukin-6 157
intermittent fasting 117–19, 166
International Space Station 122
inulin 158, 159
iron in food 150
irritability 37
Jacka, Prof Felice 142, 149–52
Jerusalem artichokes 159
  beef and Jerusalem artichoke casserole
    260–1
  Jerusalem artichoke soup 231–2
jet lag 72–8, 125
journals 123–4
junk food 52, 63, 82, 92, 148, 155, 195

kale: mushroom, chickpea and kale curry
    266–7
kimchi 164
  scrambled eggs with kimchi 227
  tofu, leek and kimchi broth 235–6
kiwi fruit 143
Kleitman, Prof Nathaniel 90

laboratory tests 91, 104, 148
Lactobacillus 155, 163, 165
lamb: meatballs with feta and eggplant
    264–6
  shepherd's pie with parsnip and white
    bean mash 269–70
larks 48, 50–4, 81, 114, 134–5, 137
lavender 128–9
leaky gut syndrome 119
leeks 158
  tofu, leek and kimchi broth 235–6
legumes 14, 128
lentils 97, 158, 162–3
  curried lentil soup with turmeric 236–7
  shepherd's pie with parsnip and white
    bean mash 269–70
  turkey and lentil Bolognese 272–3
leptin 176
light 213
  blue light 116, 121–2
  circadian clock 48, 55, 57, 71, 72
  daylight 122
  dimming lights 121–2
  morning exposure 136–7, 183
light boxes 82, 136–7, 173
light bulbs 17, 178
light sleep 21, 22–3
Lincoln, Abraham 172
liver: biological clock 49
  caffeine and the 46
  synthetic melatonin 126
Loewi, Otto 32–3

lorry drivers 62
lunges 200

M score 142, 145–6, 184, 203, 212
Maas, James 138
McCartney, Paul 32
mackerel: baked sweet potato with
    smoked mackerel 240
  mackerel, beetroot and tahini pitta
    251–2
magnesium supplements 128
mattresses 178
meal times 49, 118, 137–8, 139, 166, 214
measurements before beginning
    programme 176–7
meatballs with feta and eggplant 264–6
medication: caffeine processing effects 46
  melatonin 74, 84, 125–6, 130, 173
  microbiome diversity 155
  parasomnia 68
  sleeping pills 74, 85–6, 125–7
meditation 130–1
Mediterranean diet 142, 144–52, 184,
    220, 223, 276
melatonin 84, 130, 137, 213
  cherries 143
  daily cycle 49, 55, 57, 116, 121
  function 125
  jet lag reduction 74
  shift work 84
  supplements 74, 125–6, 173
memory: ageing and 28–9
  cytokines 157
  deep sleep and 3, 25–6, 27–9
  jet lag and 73
  poor sleep effects 2
  short-term and long-term 27–8
men, sleep and gender differences 42
menopause 94–8
metabolic syndrome 36–7

microbiome 203
  ageing and the 94
  diet effects 149, 153, 178, 213, 215, 223
  diversity 154–6
  effect on sleep 141–2, 215
  IBS 165
  overview 112–13, 152–4
  poor sleep effects 2
  prebiotics 157–63
  testing 155–6
mind, slowing down a racing 206–9
mindfulness 204, 207, 208–9, 213–14,
    216
mobile phones 116, 121–2, 179, 182
modafinil 85–6
ModiMed diet 150–2
monitoring sleep 39–42, 172–3
mood: Mediterranean diet and 149–52
  and the microbiome 112, 154
  poor sleep effects 37
  and probiotics 165
  REM sleep 29–31
  Sleep Restriction Therapy (SRT) 190,
    192
Mosley, Dr Michael: insomnia 2, 4, 57–8,
    59–60, 130
  sleep deprivation experience 102–4
muffins: sweet potato savoury muffins
    with feta 228–9
Multiple Sleep Latency Test 91
muscles: muscle paralysis 29
  muscle relaxation 207–8
  muscle twitches 23
mushrooms: chicken noodles with pak
    choi 234–5
  mushroom, chickpea and kale curry
    266–7
  ratatouille with white beans 267–8
  shepherd's pie with parsnip and white
    bean mash 269–70

super-speedy mushroom risotto with
  edamame 246–7
turkey and lentil Bolognese 272–3
music 123, 130, 178, 213
Musk, Elon 117, 135

naps: evenings 111
  jet lag 78
  long car journeys 106–7
  not during SRT 188
  shift work 80, 81, 82, 83
  siestas 58, 138
narcolepsy 85
National Sleep Foundation 87–8, 123,
  179
neck size and snoring 61, 63–4, 176,
  215
Nedergaard, Dr Maiken 120–1
negative thinking 132, 202, 206–7
nervous system 131
nervousness 30
neurons 23, 32–3
nightmares 67, 143–4
noodles: chicken noodles with pak choi
  234–5
  tofu, leek and kimchi broth 235–6
nori 161
  nori chilli popcorn 255–6
  nori-flavoured warm salmon and
    butternut pumpkin salad 273–5
  nori rolled crab 254–5
nuts 128, 163, 212
  nutty berry crunch 287–8
  oaty nutty shake 225
  see also almonds; walnuts, etc

oats 15, 184
  nutty berry crunch 287–8
  oaty nutty shake 225
  rosy overnight oats 226

obesity: effect on sleep 35–6, 147
  sleep deprivation 33–6
Obstructive Sleep Apnoea (OSA) 61–5,
  94
oestrogen 37, 94, 95
onions 158
  baked turmeric-spiced fennel and onion
    276–7
  fermented fennel and onion 291–2
  purple pickled onions 186, 290–1
oranges: zucchini, orange and apricot cake
  286–7
orgasms 39
orthosomnia 40
OSA (Obstructive Sleep Apnoea) 61–5,
  94
owls 48, 50–6, 81, 114
oxidative stress 152
oxytocin 37

pak choi, chicken noodles with 234–5
pancreas 118
Panda, Dr Satchin 117, 118, 119
paradoxical intention 207
parasomnia 3–4, 67–9
parasympathetic system 131
parsnips: shepherd's pie with parsnip and
    white bean mash 269–70
pasta: hot-smoked salmon, anchovies,
    artichoke and broccoli pasta 244–5
  pasta with peas and goat's cheese 242–3
  turkey and lentil Bolognese 272–3
Pavlov, Ivan 130
Peake, Tim 122
peas: pasta with peas and goat's cheese
  242–3
  smokey fish gratin 270–1
peptide YY 96
phobias 30–1
pickled onions, purple 290–1

pillows 179
pine nuts: griddled eggplant with feta and
    pine nuts 241–2
pineal gland 121, 125
Piriton 127–8
pitta, mackerel, beetroot and tahini
    251–2
Pittsburgh Sleep Quality Index 89, 147
pituitary gland 23
plank exercise 200
poo 152, 155–6
popcorn, nori chilli 255–6
porridge 97, 159
positive thinking 133
pranayama 130–1, 185, 207–8
prawns and red cabbage slaw on
    sourdough 250–1
prayer 124
prebiotics 157–63
prediabetes 176
prefrontal cortex 28, 29
pregnancy 126, 127, 164, 172
primates, quantity of sleep 98–9
prions 100
probiotics 163–5
problem solving 31–3
Progressive Muscle Relaxation 204, 207–8
prosciutto, baked chicory with 238
protein 119, 141, 158
    increasing 94–8
psychobiotics 153
puberty 52
push-ups 199

quality of sleep: and body fat 35–6
    food and 8, 141–2, 147–9
    microbiome diversity 154–6
    probiotics 165
quantity of sleep: evolution 98–9
    recommended 87–8

tests 89–91
    time in bed compared to actual sleep 89
questionnaires: insomnia 109–10
    larks and owls 51
    M score 145–6
    Pittsburgh Sleep Quality Index 89, 147
quinoa 97

radicchio 158
ratatouille with white beans 267–8
Raubenheimer, Prof David 94
raw food diet 104
reaction times, sleep deprivation and 102,
    103
Rechtschaffen, Allan 99
relaxation 207–8
REM (Rapid Eye Movement) sleep
    19–20, 21, 29–30
research: adjusting circadian clock 55–6
    ageing 28–9
    alcohol 120–1
    Bimuno 161–3
    brain alertness in sleep 104
    children 35, 52, 53–4
    chronotypes 52
    clock changes 107–8
    depression 142, 149–51, 192
    EEG monitoring 18–20
    exercise 197–8
    food 141–2, 144, 147–8, 149–52, 164,
        165
    HRT 98
    jet lag 73, 74
    melatonin 74, 126
    memory 28–59, 157
    microbiome 156
    new parents 92–3
    protein and hunger 95, 96
    school start time 53
    sex 37–9

shift work 79, 81, 83, 84
short-sleep mutations 105
sleep deprivation 33–9, 99
sleep patterns 58–9
sleep quantity 88
Sleep Restriction Therapy (SRT) 190–2
sleeping while driving 106
time-restricted eating (TRE) 166
weight gain 33–6
resistance exercise 135, 185, 199–201, 204, 205
rewards 35
rice: nori rolled crab 254–5
super-speedy mushroom risotto with edamame 246–7
Richards, Keith 32
ricotta: cashew, ricotta and red capsicum dip 249–50
Roiter, Dr Ignazio 100–1
routines: bedtime 117–25, 205
exercise 135, 199–201
extreme larks 134
wake-up-go-to-bed 114
waking 134

SAD (Seasonal Affective Disorder) 136–7
salads: black bean salad with lime and avocado 252–3
Dr Tim's hot-smoked salmon salad 239
nori-flavoured warm salmon and butternut pumpkin salad 273–5
red cabbage slaw 250–1
seeded rainbow salad 279–80
tabbouleh with goat's cheese 256–7
salmon: Dr Tim's hot-smoked salmon salad 239
hot-smoked salmon, anchovies, artichoke and broccoli pasta 244–5
nori-flavoured warm salmon and butternut pumpkin salad 273–5

sardines on seeded sourdough 245
sauerkraut 164, 178
school start time 53, 92
SCN (suprachiasmatic nucleus) 48–9, 125
Scott, Eleanor 33, 34
Seasonal Affective Disorder (SAD) 136–7
seaweed see nori
'second sleep' 58–9, 60
serotonin 112, 154, 156, 203
sex drive 37–9
sexsomnia 67
Shelley, Mary 32
shepherd's pie with parsnip and white bean mash 269–70
shift work 3, 70–2, 78–86, 114, 138
Shift Work Sleep Disorder (SWSD) 84–5
showers 123
siestas 58, 138
Simpson, Prof Steve 94
sleep: recommended amount 87–108
science of 15–167
stages of 21–4
ways to improve 109–40
what keeps us awake 57–86
what puts us to sleep 45–56
why we need so much 98–9
sleep apnoea 36, 61–6, 79
sleep deprivation: euphoria during 103
Fatal Familial Insomnia (FFI) 100–1
how long you can stay awake 99–105
Michael's experience 102–4
older people 93–4
parents 92–3
records 101–2
research 33–9, 99
shift work 70–2
teenagers 52, 53–4, 92, 116
women 42

sleep drive 111, 115
sleep eating 24, 67, 68
sleep efficiency: calculation 41–2, 172–3
   diet 147–9, 157, 152–3
   genes 46–7, 50–1
   insomnia 189, 191
   target 7, 172–3
sleep hygiene 112, 113, 178–80, 181–2,
      185, 194, 198
sleep inertia 138
sleep laboratories 91, 104, 148
sleep mutants 105
Sleep Onset Latency Test 89–91
sleep patterns: pre-industrial 58–9, 71–2,
      133
research 58–9
Sleep Restriction Therapy (SRT): benefits
      192
   how to do it 187–92
   introduction to 9–10, 111–13
   method 181–92
   preparation 171–220
   week 1 181–92, 218
   week 2 193–201, 218
   week 3 202–11, 219
   week 4 212–17, 219
'sleep start' 23
sleep talking 24, 67
sleep tracking 39–43, 173
sleep window 114, 214
sleepiness, lack of at bedtime 129
sleeping pills 74, 125–8, 130
sleepwalking 24, 66–9
snacks 14, 118–19, 195, 244, 283
snoring 60–6
   and ageing 93–4
   alcohol and 120
   anti-snoring devices 66
   menopause 94
   neck size and 61, 63–4, 176, 215

records 61
   and sleep apnoea 61–5
   surgery 66
   weight and 35, 61, 63–5
social jet lag 49, 115
social media 116
soups: anti-inflammatory Chinese-style
      chicken broth 233–4
   cauliflower and roasted red capsicum
      soup 230–1
   chicken noodles with pak choi 234–5
   curried lentil soup with turmeric 236–7
   Jerusalem artichoke soup 231–2
   tofu, leek and kimchi broth 235–6
spiders 31
Spielman, Arthur 191–2
spinach: Dr Tim's hot-smoked salmon
      salad 239
   nori-flavoured warm salmon and
      butternut pumpkin salad 273–5
   spinach in garlic yoghurt 281–2
   tabbouleh with goat's cheese 256–7
Spoon Test 89–91
squats 200
Stead, Tim 208–9
stimulus control 129–30, 203
'Stone Age' diet 104
stress 23, 35, 176, 215, 219–20
studying 28, 85
sugar 14, 34–5, 141, 195
sunlight 48
supplements 128, 161–3, 165, 173
suprachiasmatic nucleus (SCN) 48–9,
      125
surgery for snoring 66
sweet potatoes: baked sweet potato with
      smoked mackerel 240
   sweet potato savoury muffins with feta
      228–9
Syndrome X 36–7

tabbouleh with goat's cheese 256–7

tagine: chicken tagine with chickpeas and dates 263–4

tahini: mackerel, beetroot and tahini pitta 251–2

tau protein 25

teenagers 2–3, 52–54, 88, 92, 116

telepathy 18–19

television 116, 178, 190

temperature, body 22, 49, 118, 123

temptation removal 115–16, 178–9, 181–2

testosterone 37

thalamus 100

Thatcher, Margaret 1

thought challenges 131–2, 202, 206

throats, snoring 61

time-restricted eating (TRE) 177, 183–4, 194, 213
   benefits of 117–18, 119
   method 118–19, 166
   shift work 79, 80, 81

'to-do' journal 123–4, 184

tofu 97
   leek and kimchi broth 235–6

toilet trips 57–8, 133

tomatoes: meatballs with feta and eggplant 264–6
   ratatouille with white beans 267–8
   turkey and lentil Bolognese 272–3

toxins in the brain 25

tracking sleep 39–42, 173

'transcranial direct current stimulation' 29

triceps dip 200–1

trout with celeriac mash 258–9

truck drivers 63

tryptophan 128, 143

turkey: tryptophan myth 142–3

turkey and lentil Bolognese 272–3

UK SLEEP CENSUS 88–9

urination 57–8, 133

uvula 61

uvulopalatopharyngoplasty 66

valerian 128

vegetables: chicken and veg tray bake 262–3
   fermented vegetables 289–92
   nutrition 128, 276
   roasted vegetables with thyme 278–9
   see also individual types of vegetable

vicious circle, sleep and weight gain 35–6

vitamins: B vitamins 158

vitamin B12 150

vitamin K 153

Wahlberg, Mark 134

waist measurement 176–7, 215, 220, 223

wake-up-go-to-bed routine 114

waking: at night 57–8, 59–60, 130, 132–35
   hormones 45
   routine 134

wake-up time 181, 183

walking 136, 183, 204, 217

walnuts: banana on toast with crunchy walnuts 285
   braised red cabbage with walnuts and apple 277–8

weekend lie-ins 114–115, 186

Wehr, Dr Thomas 58–9

weight: measuring before the programme 176–7

weight gain: effect on sleep 35–6
   menopause and 94
   sleep deprivation 2, 33–38
   and snoring 61

weight loss: Sleep Restriction Therapy (SRT) 215–16

and snoring reduction 63–65
  time restricted eating (TRE) 166
  weight loss vs sleep improvement 177
wholegrains 159
willpower 199
wine 120, 121
women: menopause 94–8
  shift work 84
  sleep and gender differences 42
worrying 124, 129, 131–2, 184, 203, 206
Worthman, Carol 59
Wright, Dr Kenneth 56
Wright, Tony 102–4, 105

yoghurt 97, 163
  black grapes with yoghurt and almonds
    224–5
  celery with blue cheese dip 248–9
  rosy overnight oats 226
  smoked mackerel, beetroot and tahini
    pitta 251–2
  spinach in garlic yoghurt 281–2
yogic breathing 130–1, 185, 207–8

zoplicone 74, 125, 126–7
zucchini, orange and apricot cake 286–7
Zuckerberg, Mark 135

Acknowledgements

A big thanks to my niece, Emily, for producing the charming and witty drawings for this book. They still make me smile! I would also like to thank all those who shared their sleep stories with me and the numerous academics who shared their knowledge and expertise. And finally a big thank you to Aurea and Rebecca who have provided so much help and support since my first book, *The Fast Diet*.

Dr Michael Mosley is a science presenter, journalist and executive producer. After training to be a doctor at the Royal Free Hospital in London, he spent 25 years at the BBC, where he made numerous science documentaries. Now freelance, he is the author of several best-selling books, *The Fast Diet*, *The 8-Week Blood Sugar Diet*, *The Clever Guts Diet*, *The Fast 800*, *The Fast Keto* and *Just One Thing*. He is married with four children.
Instagram: @michaelmosley_official

Dr Clare Bailey, wife of Michael Mosley, is a GP who has pioneered a dietary approach to health and reducing blood sugars and diabetes at her surgery in Buckinghamshire. She is the author of *The 8-Week Blood Sugar Diet Recipe Book*, *The Clever Guts Diet Recipe Book*, *The Fast 800 Recipe Book*, *The Fast 800 Easy* and *The Fast 800 Keto Recipe Book*.
Instagram: @drclarebailey

Justine Pattison is one of the UK's leading healthy-eating recipe writers. She has published numerous books, makes regular appearances on television, can often be heard on the radio and contributes to many top magazines, newspapers and websites.
Website: www.justinepattison.com